Recipes to the Rescue

Recipes to the Rescue

Lindy Kingsmill

Jann Bonner

Suzanne Morrow

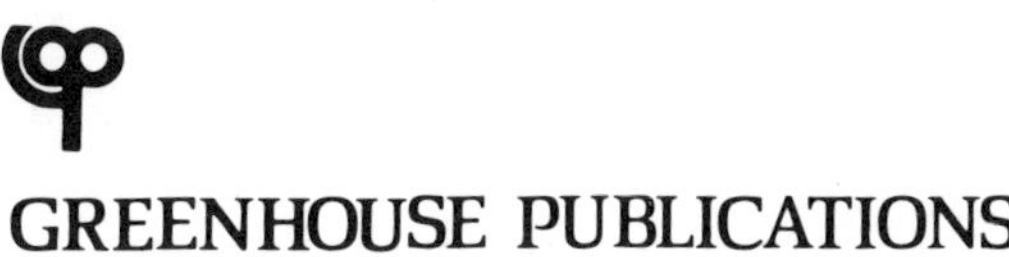

GREENHOUSE PUBLICATIONS

First published in 1988 by
Greenhouse Publications Pty Ltd
385-387 Bridge Road
Richmond Victoria Australia 3121

© Jann Bonner Lindy Kingsmill Suzanne Morrow 1988

Photography Phil Wymant Latrobe Studios Melbourne
Food stylist Ann Creber
Design Tom Kurema

Typeset by Dead Set Fitzroy Victoria
Printed and bound by
Kyodo-Shing Loong Singapore

National Library of Australia
Cataloguing-in-Publication data
Bonner, Jann
   Recipes to the rescue.

   ISBN 0 86436 125 4.

   1. Food allergy – Diet therapy – Recipes.
   I. Kingsmill, Lindy. II. Morrow, Suzanne.
   III. Title.

641.5'631

*Front cover: Lentil and Walnut Pâté, Icecreams, Lemon Meringue Pie and
a glass of apple juice*

Back cover: Peanut Butter Cake, and Avocado Soup and Seed Bread

TABLE OF CONTENTS

FOREWORD

In the last ten years milk allergy, lactose intolerance, gluten sensitivity, Candida Albicans, hyperactivity, rheumatism/arthritis and reactivity to mould and fungus have become familiar terms to many Australians who have gained a great deal of relief from their varied allergenic and food reactive symptoms by restricting certain foods in their diets. After realising that the dietary changes really help contribute to wellness, there is usually a period of transition when finding the right foods can be a problem.

There *is* plenty to eat — it's just a matter of finding new foods. However, this is not so easy and many do need help. A cookbook and dietary guide containing recipes that work with suitable substitutes has for a long time been needed, and so often books are presented on allergy food substitutes with inadequate thought to the total restriction of offending foods.

If a patient is, therefore, to be put on such a diet, it is important that all allergenic foods be totally avoided for a period of time until noticeable improvement occurs. Then a challenge with the offending food can be tried. During such periods help is most definitely needed in the kitchen.

Recipes to the Rescue is an excellent book for allergy sufferers as it gives guidelines for healthy eating, planned menus, and is presented in a common sense manner. The authors are women with allergies themselves and with allergenic children and they know what it is like to feed hungry families. They have been working with allergy diets for a number of years, and show you how to make the best dietary contribution to your family's wellbeing through the right choice of foods.

Recipes to the Rescue gives many substitutes, the food tastes good and the alternatives work. I know this book will be a great asset to patient and practitioner alike.

Maureen Baranski, ND DMH
Clinical Ecologist, Naturopath,
Herbalist, Nutritionist.
Wahroonga, Sydney, 1987.

ACKNOWLEDGEMENT

We would like to express our appreciation to Helen Bracher for her contribution to this book.

INTRODUCTION

Increasing numbers of us today are looking beyond our Western diet with its heavy overload of processed foods, salt, sugar, fats and animal protein, toward a healthier style of eating; a dietary pattern which emphasises natural and unprocessed foods with an abundance of fresh fruits and vegetables, complemented by wholegrains, nuts and seeds. The transition is not always easy.

For those of us in the kitchen, the daily preparation of meals can become an exacting task, particularly when we decide to change our style of eating because of the challenge of illness or food intolerance, or because we are becoming increasingly aware that we and our families can lead fuller and more meaningful lives if we are fit and healthy. This is everyone's birthright and the foundation of it is the food we eat — the food we select, prepare and serve on the family table. So when confronted with the challenge of achieving this by reducing or eliminating familiar foods and substituting new and unfamiliar ones, the preparation of food to nourish and please a critical family can seem an insurmountable problem. We may well feel like slipping back to our old ways or stocking up again from the supermarket. With patience and perseverance the battle can be won and a revolution achieved in our own kitchens.

This book was written to assist in just such a situation and is the work of three friends who, when faced with food allergies and illness in their own families, set about radically changing their eating habits. The recipes are based on a natural diet, high in fresh fruits and vegetables, wholegrains, nuts and seeds, low in salt and fat. They totally exclude sugar, artificial additives and overly processed foods. For those struggling with food allergies and searching for recipes both suitable and tasty, the great majority of them either exclude the major allergens or can be adapted to do so.

The recipes are a result of several years research, discussion and experimentation. They are designed specifically for those attempting to follow a healthy eating pattern whilst coping with food intolerance. However, you don't have to be allergic to anything to enjoy and benefit from these recipes. They are nutritious, they do exclude foods which may be harmful, but first and foremost we think they're delicious. It is our sincere wish that you will too.

Good cooking and bon appetit.

ABOUT ALLERGY

The case histories included here are typical examples of the variety of symptoms experienced by allergy sufferers and the treatments which lead to improvement.

M.S. Cow's milk allergy from childhood. After first pregnancy occurrence of multiple allergies to goat's milk, yeast, soy and grains causing depression, lethargy, arthritis, headache and bleeding from bowel. With herbal and homeopathic treatment, vitamin and mineral supplements and restriction and rotation of foods, there has been a gradual return to tolerating small amounts of most foods.

A.E. Cow's milk, egg, soy, yeast and grain allergies from early childhood led to variety of physical and mental symptoms — vomiting, stomach ache, timidity, fear attacks and frequent colds and infections. Repeated courses of antibiotics to no effect. Homeopathy, rotation of foods, and mineral and vitamin supplementation led to immediate improvement and gradual tolerance of most foods.

E.B. Mucous, vomiting and sleeplessness at birth and early months due to yeast allergy through mother. With removal of yeast no symptoms present.

A.K. Abdominal pain and genital itching. Allergen found to be yeast. Complete improvement with elimination. After some time, now tolerates yeast three times a week without any problems.

M.J. Nausea, irritable and bubbly stomach, flatulence, thrush, frequent colds, sinusitis, tiredness. Fourteen allergies detected. Complete improvement in six to twelve weeks. The most persistent allergen, being yeast, disappeared after introducing yoghurt and apple cider vinegar to the diet (not commonly considered a cure for yeast allergy, but helpful for some people). Now able to tolerate yeast two or three times per week.

A.J. Avoidance of dairy products and other allergens by mother during third pregnancy. Baby totally breast fed for ten months before introduction of solids. Result — very healthy and no allergies to date. Except for some yoghurt, dairy products are still excluded.

L.L. Suffered during childhood from tonsillitis, bronchitis and other infections. Repeated courses of antibiotics. Health improved since eliminating junk foods and cow's milk. Vitamin and mineral supplementation has helped. No longer suffers from respiratory infections.

Food sensitivities occur with distressing frequency throughout the population and can range from a mild intolerance to a single food causing little inconvenience to debilitating allergies to multiple foods and substances. Drs J. and B. Rudolph[1] estimate that 100 million people in the USA have an allergy of some sort and that one-fifth or 20 per cent of those require expert medical care. These percentages are relevant to Australia today. In addition, of course, there are many people visiting their doctors repeatedly with allergy-induced symptoms whose causes are not recognised and thus not adequately treated.

It is tempting to see this problem as a modern phenomenon, and indeed it is in the size and complexity of it. However, such conditions have been recorded throughout the ages; as long ago as 3000 BC in China; in Egyptian hieroglyphics; by Hippocrates who was aware that people suffering from headache should not be given milk, and by Lucretius in the first century BC who must have been referring to allergy when he said — 'one man's meat is another man's poison'.

So food intolerances appear far back in the history of mankind, but it would seem today that an increasing proportion of the population is falling prey to these problems. This requires some explanation. There is little doubt that the cause lies in our increasingly devitalised and chemically contaminated food supply; the excessive, and often unnecessary, use of antibiotics which destroys vital bacteria in the bowel and lays the foundation for faulty absorption of valuable nutrients; and the poisoning of our air, water and soil with dangerous chemicals.

Allergy based illnesses occur because the body is unable to cope with such an onslaught, and the result is a lowered immune response. These conditions present via a variety of symptoms, some of which are listed below.

Some symtoms that have been found to be caused by allergies:

Muscular — joint stiffness, arthritis, joint pains, muscle cramps or spasms, muscle weakness, aching.

Genitourinary — frequent urination, painful or difficult urination, bedwetting, genital itch.

Headaches — various kinds including migraine.

Mental-behavioural — anxiety, depression, agitation, erratic behaviour, irritability, tension, crying, schizophrenia.

Respiratory — coughing, asthma, wheezing, hayfever, 'frequent colds', chronic rhinitis, nosebleeds, postnasal discharge, sinusitis, sore throat, mouth breathing, enlarged tonsils and adenoids.

Ear — hearing loss, infections, ringing in the ear, inflammation, sensation of fullness or blocking.

Skin — itching, hives, rashes, pallor, acne, eczema, dermatitis.

Cardiovascular — rapid or slowed pulse, chest pain, high or low blood pressure.

---

1. Allergies: What they are and what to do about them. See Bibliography.

Gastrointestinal — nausea, vomiting, spastic colon, bloatedness, flatulence, diarrhoea, constipation, heartburn, gall bladder pains, gastro-intestinal bleeding.

Central nervous system — fatigue, hyperactivity, insomnia, nightmares, dizziness, convulsions, sensation of imbalance, learning disorders, poor concentration, poor muscle coordination.

Eye — blurred vision, itching, burning, conjunctivitis, sensitivity to light.

Other — abnormal body odour, dark circles under the eyes, hypoglycaemia, diabetes, excessive sweating.

Allergists tell us that allergies run in families. A child born into a family with a number of allergy-prone members has a greater probability of developing allergies than one in a family with fewer allergy-prone members. Through the study of the family tree, certain patterns such as the frequency of a particular illness, can become apparent. Some allergists believe that allergy is one factor in the development of these illnesses and that successful treatment of the allergy may control or even prevent them.[2]

Another very important factor involved in the predisposition to allergies is exposure to foreign proteins such as cow's milk and gluten during the first year of life. Allergic reactions are caused because of the lack of enzymes necessary to digest these foods. For this reason complementary feeds given in hospital can have a detrimental effect on a baby's immature digestive system and can be a major cause of colic. Breast fed babies can also be affected by the mother drinking milk. It is often said that cow's or goat's milk are good foods for baby cows or baby goats but inappropriate for humans, being difficult to digest and often causing mucous problems and allergies in susceptible people. Those unable to tolerate milk may be able to tolerate a little yoghurt and home-made cottage cheese as these are pre-digested and more easily assimilated. It must be remembered however, that each person is an individual with an individual response.

Many practitioners send their patients to an allergist to detect the substances to which they are allergic. This is usually done by means of a RAST blood test. The advantage of this is that from one sample of blood many substances can be tested without the person experiencing unpleasant side effects. The disadvantage is that it is expensive and it may not detect all the allergens to which the person is sensitive.

Another test commonly done is a provocative test where a substance is given sublingually (under the tongue) or intradermally (under the skin) in order to provoke a response. If the person is sensitive he or she will usually respond with an allergic symptom.

Other tests for the detection of food allergens can be inexpensive and some can be performed by the patient, perhaps with guidance from a practitioner. The Coca pulse test is based on the idea that the pulse be-

---

2. Reading C and Meillon R; *Relatively Speaking*, Fontana Australia 1981.

comes substantially elevated after contact with or ingestion of an allergen. It can be conducted in the home by the patients themselves over a period of time.[3]

Muscle weakness is an indicator of allergic reaction. Tests can be conducted for this in the home. They are simple and cost nothing, but are not infallible.[4]

Elimination diets are probably the most reliable means of testing allergens. Suspect foods and substances are eliminated from the diet, then reintroduced individually after a period of time. The reaction to these foods is observed. This can be a slow process and is best if supervised by a practitioner.

Many people have successfully treated their allergy problems using a variety of methods including elimination and rotation diets, raw food diets, the use of natural therapies such as herbs and homeopathy, relaxation and reflexology, and vitamin and mineral supplementation. The bibliography lists a number of books which will be of great assistance in this process. We wish you well in your efforts to overcome these distressing problems. Results *can* be obtained quickly although often it is a slow process, but patience and perseverance will be rewarded.

3.   Coca, Arthur F: *The Pulse Test*, New York. Arco Publishing Company, Inc.
4.   Baker Elton & Elizabeth: *The Uncook Book*, Colorado. Drelwood Publications.

ALLERGY DIETS

Just about everyone knows how difficult it can be to stay on a diet whether it's to avoid allergens or to slim. Those wonderful resolutions, which seem so easy before we start, filling us with zeal and determination, can waver and crumble after a few days without our favourite foods.

Staying on the diet may appear to be a life sentence and if allergens are your problem, one with hard labour. There is no escaping the fact that if you, or a family member, are suffering from food allergies then you are going to spend a fair bit of time in the kitchen preparing food. Although the range of prepared substitute foods available in health shops is increasing, it is still economically and in the interests of health, better to do it yourself. Not that the range of natural substitute biscuits, crispbreads and noodles is not useful, but the homecooking of breads, cookies and cakes is the preferable, and often the only way, of having them. Below are five steps to assist you to keep to the diet, so that you don't find yourself faced with an empty pantry, saying 'What the heck', and slipping up to the local shop for a loaf of bread or a packet of biscuits.

Motivation This of course is the basis of all endeavours whatever their purpose. In following an allergy diet remember how you felt before you removed or reduced that food or foods, remember headaches, weight problems, arthritis, hayfever, sinus, stomach disorders and remind yourself that you are feeling better than you have felt in a long time, that you are building your body and mind toward better health and, with that, preventing the onset of more serious disease.

So, think positive.

Planning Planning your family menu a week or a fortnight ahead, will enable you to get through the period smoothly. It means you can make the most of the foods available to you, in terms of variety, and if necessary the rotation of allergens. It also means that during the arsenic hours between 5 pm and 7 pm you won't arrive home and wonder how on earth you can get a sensible, nutritionally-based, allergy-planned and delicious meal on the table in half an hour.

So, plan your menus ahead.

Preparation

Once you've planned your menu, taking into account foods in season and those which can be refrigerated, and the late nights home or early meals, then you need to ensure you have your cupboards stocked. Regular weekly or fortnightly checks before shopping will mean that you don't run out of much needed items such as rice flour, soy milk or agar flakes, just when you need them. This sort of organisation is really no different to that needed for a normal diet, except that most of these 'substitute items' are only available at good health food shops which may be some distance away. For most of us with allergies there is no popping up to the corner shop at the last minute for a necessary item.

So, prepare in advance.

Organisation

You need to keep an eye on your menu plan a day or so ahead. Many dishes, for example jellies or legumes, require advance preparation involving soaking or pre-cooking. The whole week's balance can be thrown out if you plan Lentil Shepherd's Pie with rice and Strawberry Jelly Mould for dinner but have forgotten to cook the lentils and soak the agar. It is an excellent idea to set aside 15-30 minutes daily, perhaps after dinner before doing the dishes, not only for this sort of organisation but also to prepare a cake, a batch of biscuits, cookies or fruit balls to have 'in the tin'. Looking ahead is important for perseverance on allergy diets.

Perseverance

Knowing that the diet is working well for you is an enormous incentive to continue. Having the recipes, foods and menu plans organised is another. However, with all that it isn't easy to give up our favourite foods to maintain the diet when eating away from home. So if you slip occasionally, enjoy it and forget it. Get back to the foods you know work well for you and keep on with them. You'll find that if you follow the above steps, apart from the moments of sheer indulgence or those that are unavoidable, the path of the allergy diet will be fairly smooth for you. It also helps to know that you are doing much to promote optimum health in yourself and your family.

So, persevere regardless.

The following menu plans for a week are examples of how you can plan a diet around food intolerances. Of course not all members of a family will be allergic to anything or even the same thing. This is where you need to consult a practitioner experienced in this field. One, to determine the extent of the allergy and two, to assist you in planning the best ways to overcome it, be it total exclusion of the food(s) or rotation of it (them) over a set period.

A list of books has been included which will provide you with a wide range of information, from all over the world, on the methods used to diagnose and treat food intolerance. We urge you to read as widely as you can, because even with the best advice and treatment it is still up to you to overcome your problem.

The basic aim of these menus is to provide you with a nutritious balance and a variety of foods while making the appropriate elimination or rotations. It is up to you to work out your individual plan in consultation with your nutritionally oriented allergy practitioner.

Finally, after you have done all this thinking, planning, organising and cooking, don't expect your family to say thank you all at once. It can be very discouraging indeed to have done all this, a major achievement in itself, and to have your labours greeted with looks of disbelief and complaints about the food. Don't panic and don't give up!

From experience we can say two things:

Persevere; ensure that you are not in a halfway situation, e.g. half white flour and sugar, and half the diet you are trying to encourage. It is often very difficult to get some children to eat whole grains or honey when they know if they hold out they can still have sugary biscuits, potato chips and commercial icecream. It is far better to exclude such foods from the pantry altogether.

Remain calm and don't insist that an unpopular food is eaten, but reintroduce it after an interval of a couple of weeks. You will find that more and more foods will be accepted and may well become favourites.

SUMMER MENU PLAN

Sunday

Breakfast	*Lunch*	*Dinner*
fresh fruit, nuts and/or seeds OR Sunshine Breakfast	sesame fish, baked potato or sweet potato and tossed salad OR carrot and nut loaf, baked potato or sweet potato and salad fruit salad with cashew cream	*tofu, salad, nori and sprouts with Ryvita biscuits OR buckwheat pancakes with stewed or freshly grated apple

Monday

muesli made from puffed millet or soaked rolled millet, ground nuts and seeds with nut milk fresh fruit if desired	avocado, salad and sprouts, millet waffles or millet muffins	chicken and almonds and salad or steamed vegies OR hiziki pie with steamed vegies or salad. strawberry jelly OR layered fruit salad with strawberry sauce

Tuesday

fresh fruit nuts and/or seeds	hummus on rice cakes with salad and toasted nori	fried rice with roasted nuts tossed salad or steamed vegies fruit jelly or fruit in season

Wednesday

Breakfast	Lunch	Dinner
buckwheat pancakes with fresh pear OR fresh fruit with nuts and seeds	*tofu with salad and sprouts or sardine spread with salad and sprouts OR lentil pâté with salad and sprouts and buckwheat crispbread	vegetarian rolls tossed salad, sprouts OR *tofu casserole with salad or steamed vegies cream caramel OR carob ice cream with fruit

Thursday

Breakfast	Lunch	Dinner
fresh fruit with breakfast sprinkle OR muesli made from puffed millet or soaked millet, ground nuts and seeds with nut milk and fresh fruit	millet muffins or millet waffles with date seed spread, salad and sprouts OR Ryvita biscuits with date seed spread, salad and sprouts	sesame chicken steamed sweet potato, salad and steamed vegies OR vegetable crumble with tossed salad fresh fruit OR apple pie

Friday

Breakfast	Lunch	Dinner
sesame rice waffles with nut butter or tahini or berry jam OR brown rice muesli	rice cakes with tahini or nut butter, salad and sprouts OR rice salad, tossed salad and sunflower seeds or pepitas	baked whole schnapper with tossed salad or steamed vegies OR potato pancakes with tossed salad or steamed vegies fresh fruit salad

Saturday

Breakfast	Lunch	Dinner
fresh fruit nuts and/or seeds OR barley waffles with berry jam	avocado, corn on the cob, salad and sprouts OR corn fritters, salad and sprouts	lentil shepherd's pie with mashed pumpkin topping tossed salad or steamed vegies. fresh fruit in season

Drinks — cold lemon grass tea, herb teas, vegetable juices, diluted fruit juice, smoothies

Snacks — frozen treats, crudites, muffins, scones, crackers and crispbreads, seeds and nuts, biscuits

*Tofu is considered by some people to contain yeast. However, it seems to be well tolerated by most people with a yeast allergy.

WINTER MENU PLAN

Sunday

Breakfast	Lunch	Dinner
buckwheat porridge with nut milk and fresh pear or fresh fruit, nuts and/or seeds	sesame fish, baked potato or sweet potato and steamed vegies OR carrot and nut loaf, baked potato or sweet potato and steamed vegetables fruit salad with cashew cream	vegetable soup *tofu salad, nori and sprouts with Ryvita biscuits OR buckwheat pancakes with stewed or freshly grated apple

Monday

millet porridge, made from either rolled millet or organic hulled millet with nut milk and chopped banana OR millet waffles with mashed banana	pumpkin soup avocado salad and sprouts millet muffins	chicken with almonds and salad or steamed vegies OR hiziki pie with salad or steamed vegies fresh fruit in season

Tuesday

rice porridge with ground unhulled sesame seeds and sesame milk OR fresh fruit nuts and/or seeds	vegetable soup, hummus, rice cakes, salad and sprouts toasted nori	fried rice with roasted nuts and steamed vegies or tossed salad baked apples with tahini cream or fruit jelly

Wednesday

buckwheat pancakes with fresh pear OR buckwheat porridge and stewed or fresh pear	*tofu with salad and sprouts or sardine spread with salad and sprouts OR lentil pâté with salad and sprouts buckwheat crispbread	vegetarian rolls, tossed salad and sprouts OR buckwheat rissoles with steamed vegies or tossed salad

Thursday

Breakfast	Lunch	Dinner
millet porridge with nut milk and banana OR millet waffles with mashed banana	pumpkin soup millet muffins with date seed spread, salad and sprouts OR Ryvita biscuits with date seed spread, salad and sprouts	sesame chicken, sweet potato and steamed vegies or salad OR vegetable crumble with tossed salad fruit salad

Friday

Breakfast	Lunch	Dinner
sesame rice waffles with nut butter or tahini or berry jam OR rice porridge with ground sesame seeds or breakfast rice cakes	nori rolls, sprouts and salad OR rice salad, tossed salad and sunflower seeds or pepitas	vegetable soup baked whole schnapper, with steamed vegies or salad OR potato pancakes with steamed vegies or salad

Saturday

Breakfast	Lunch	Dinner
fresh fruit, nuts and/or seeds OR oat porridge and nut milk	borscht, avocado salad, sprouts and coleslaw barley waffles	lentil shepherd's pie with mashed pumpkin topping, tossed salad or steamed vegies stewed pears with carob sauce

Drinks — herb teas, dandelion coffee or some cereal coffees

Snacks — seeds and nuts, crackers, crispbreads, muffins, scones, fruit, soup

*Tofu is considered by some people to contain yeast. However it seems to be well tolerated by most people with a yeast allergy.

Additional Points

These menu plans do not adhere strictly to the food family concept. They do exclude yeast, wheat and dairy products and give alternatives to egg dishes.

Kilojoule needs vary from person to person. Additional snacks may be required by those who are very active or during growth spurts, pregnancy or lactation.

The midday meal and evening meal can be interchanged if desired.

Suggestions for meals in these menus are based on the recipes in this book.

SUBSTITUTES FOR COMMON FOODS

Dairy products Goat's milk and cheese (if tolerated).
Soy products — are useful and nutritious foods, however for some people they can be a major allergen. Soy milk is available in powdered or liquid form. We recommend that you buy a pleasant tasting liquid soy milk, for example 'Bonsoy', for making custards, sauces and for pouring on muesli and porridge. There are a few different brands in health food shops. Use powdered milk in recipes where the flavour can be disguised by other ingredients.
Tofu is a soy bean curd which may be used in some recipes as a substitute for cheese.
Nut milk — see recipe in Beverage Section.
Coconut milk — see recipes in Beverage Section.
Sesame milk — see recipe in Beverage Section.
Tahini, hummus, mashed avocado, tofu, bean spreads, lentil spreads and nut butters can be used as spreads instead of butter and margarine.

To make nut butter, grind ½-1 cup nuts in blender until ground to a fine meal. Some nuts will need no added liquid but others, for example almonds, may need a little water or cold pressed oil added to them to make a paste. How well the nuts are ground will depend on the type of blender or food processor you have.

Flours There are a number of flours available which can replace wheat and/or gluten: millet, buckwheat, brown rice, soy, polenta, potato, sweet potato, lentil, peasmeal, chick pea and arrowroot. Ground nuts and seeds can also be included in some recipes. The properties of these flours will differ from wheat flour. For example, some are crumbly because of the lack of gluten, and some work better in combination with other flours. The effectiveness of the substitute(s) will depend on the type of recipe, the other ingredients in the recipe and also to some degree on personal taste.

We have noticed that different brands of the same flour will sometimes give different results when baked, so you may find that the amount of liquid in some recipes needs to be either increased or decreased a little. The finer the flour the more liquid will be able to be absorbed. Liquid content will also vary according to weather conditions and flour moisture. Adjust the amount of liquid needed.

Breadcrumbs Replace with crushed rice cakes, ground nuts and seeds, rolled millet, grated cauliflower and cooked rice.

Pie bases Allowable flours mixed with water; ground nuts and seeds; mashed or grated vegetables for example: potato, sweet potato and pumpkin.

Tops of pies Mashed or grated vegetables; grated fruit, for example apple crumble toppings or lattice pattern made from strips of dough.

Egg Choice of an egg substitute will depend on the recipe. The following substitutes will bind in varying degrees. More than one substitute may be needed in some recipes. It is not always possible to find a good egg substitute.
Agar flakes can be used in slices and desserts.
Soy flour works well in breads, cakes, pastries and pancakes.
Tofu can be used in desserts, patties and some cakes.
Arrowroot is useful in pancakes, waffles, sauces and biscuits.
Mashed starchy vegetables can be added to loaves, patties, scones, breads and pancakes.
Mashed banana, stewed apple, pureed cooked apricots and mashed dates help to bind cakes, pancakes, scones and muffins.
Tahini, nut butters, some ground nuts, seeds and honey also help to bind.
   Some people who cannot tolerate hen eggs are sometimes able to tolerate duck, quail or turkey eggs.

Rising agents Avoid using commercial baking powder as it contains undesirable compounds including aluminium. To make baking powder, mix together 1 teaspoon bicarbonate of soda and 2 teaspoons of cream of tartar. Use approximately 1 teaspoon of this mixture for each cup of flour. Some flours may need a little extra.
   Potassium bicarbonate can be substituted for sodium bicarbonate. It is available from some chemists and health food stores and is more expensive than sodium bicarbonate, but it has the advantage of being sodium free.
   Egg whites can be beaten till stiff and folded into bread and cake mixtures to give lightness in place of baking powder.
   Use carob powder to replace cocoa as it is nutritious and contains none of the harmful alkaloids for example, caffeine and theobromine that cocoa contains.

Gelatin Use agar agar flakes to replace gelatin as it is natural, nutritious and preservative free. See Glossary for further information on agar.

HIDDEN ALLERGENS

For those who are intolerant to certain foods, we have included a list of foods that should be avoided. Often we are unaware we are eating 'forbidden foods', as it is sometimes difficult to know the content of what we are eating. Here is a rough guideline of some of the major allergens. Always check labels, but remember 'fresh is best'.

Many of these you will want to eliminate from your diet because they contain harmful substances and are not nutritious, but we have included them as a reference.

Wheat Smallgoods, sausages, devon, canned meats and fish in sauce, commercial vegetable salad, commercial thickened pie fillings, semolina, wheat breakfast cereals, some cornflours, macaroni, spaghetti, vermicelli, gravies, soups, sauces and stews thickened with wheat, malt foods, all commercial breads, baking powder, all desserts containing flour or wheat starch, ice cream cones and wafers, custard powders, packet puddings, pastry mixes, artificial cream, cream filled chocolates, pretzels, spreads and pastes, commercial sauces, relishes, chutneys, salad creams, wheat germ, beer, gin and any drink containing neutral grain spirits.

Milk Skim milk, powdered milk, buttermilk, cream, condensed milk, evaporated milk, casein, lactalbumin, lactose, butter, margarine (unless otherwise stated), curds, whey, malted milk, cheese, custards, icecream, some breads, biscuits and cakes.

Yeast Bread, biscuits, many flours are enriched with vitamins made from yeast, all cheeses especially cottage cheese, buttermilk, vinegar, most salad dressings, French dressings, tomato sauces, fermented beverages, including most alcohol beverages (brandy, beer, gin, rum, vodka, wine, whisky), most commercial sweets and desserts, malted products, mushrooms, apple cider vinegar*, mayonnaise, pickles and pickled olives, sauerkraut, horseradish, barbecue sauce, root beer, vegemite, marmite, promite, all dried fruits, antibiotics and B complex vitamins unless otherwise stated.

Fungus Moulds are present in the following and because of their close association with yeast they should also be avoided, sour cream, sour milk, yoghurt*, pumpernickel and other soured breads, pickled or smoked

---

* Some therapists are actually using these products to treat yeast sensitivity, with excellent results.

meats and fish, most sausages, hot dogs, corned beef, cider, soy sauce and all melons especially rockmelon.

Corn
Adhesives, envelopes, stamps, stickers, tapes, ale, aspirin and other tablets, bacon, baking powders, batters, beers, bleached wheat flours, whiskies, breads and pastries, breath sprays, cakes, carbonated beverages, cereals, chop suey, cornflours, cookies, corn flakes, some soy milks, commercially prepared syrups. Corn can be present in many other products from food to medical preparations.

Eggs
Some vaccines, meringues, souffles, egg sauces, cakes, biscuits, quiche, batter, pikelets, pancakes, pastry, waffles, desserts and cake mixes.

Nightshades
Tomato, capsicum, white potato and eggplant.

GUIDELINES FOR HEALTHY EATING

Foods to Avoid	Foods to Include
sugar — white, brown and raw (Read labels carefully.)	raw unheated honey, pure maple syrup, rice syrup and unsulphured dried fruit (Use sparingly for special treats.)
white flour, white rice and processed cereals	wholegrains as tolerated, especially millet and buckwheat; wholegrain flours plus soy flour, potato flour, lentil flour, peasmeal and arrowroot can be used (Grains should be either cooked or sprouted not eaten raw.)
coffee, decaffeinated coffee, tea, cola drinks, alcohol and cocoa	herb teas, vegetable juices, dandelion coffee, cereal coffee (read labels) and carob powder
cow's milk products, except perhaps a little non-fat yoghurt and cottage cheese	goat's milk (if tolerated), soy milk (if tolerated), tofu (if tolerated) nut milks and sesame milk
salt and pepper and irritating condiments	herbs, kelp powder, sea vegetables, apple cider vinegar (Small quantities of tamari and herbal seasonings may be used to flavour.)
roasted nuts and seeds (unless roasted at home without oil or salt)	unsalted raw nuts and seeds
red meat, smoked and salted fish, shellfish poultry and eggs which have been treated with chemicals, hormones and antibiotics	fresh fish, particularly deep sea fish; genuine open range poultry and eggs
fats and oils such as margarine and any oil which has been produced by using high temperatures or by chemical extraction	genuine cold pressed oils; liquid lecithin for greasing trays when baking (only a little is needed). butter, use sparingly ghee, use a little for sauteeing
all artificial colourings, preservatives, additives and flavourings tinned, processed and fast foods	fresh food as much as possible eaten raw, particularly vegetables, fruits, sprouted seeds, grains, legumes, nuts and seeds home made soups, desserts, cakes and biscuits consisting of nutritious ingredients

GLOSSARY

Some foods which appear throughout this book may be unfamiliar to you. This glossary is an easy reference.

Agar Agar Use instead of gelatin which contains sulphur dioxide (a preservative). Agar agar is made from sea vegetables and has nutritious properties, for example it is particularly rich in calcium.

The amount of agar required to gell a given quantity of liquid is affected by:

1.   The brand
The flakes used in this recipe book will make a wobbly jelly when 1 tablespoon flakes to 4 cups water is used, or a firmer jelly when 1 tablespoon flakes to 3 cups water is used.
If you are using a different brand you may need to use 2-3 times as much, as different brands of flakes have different gelling properties. It is therefore advisable to test the gelling properties of the flakes you are using e.g. by making a jelly. Agar bars and strips can also be used if preferred but again, test first.

2.   Other ingredients in the recipe
You may find some ingredients inhibit the gelling process e.g. lemon juice from some lemons, and therefore more flakes are required.

Apple Cider Vinegar Use an unpasteurised brand, preferably with the 'mother' in it, thus retaining the nutritional components. Use in salad dressings.

Arrowroot Can be used to thicken casseroles, sauces.
It is useful as a digestive aid and is actually a vegetable.

Artificial Additives Avoid these wherever possible as they are detrimental to health and may have undesirable side effects.
Always read labels.

Carob Use as an alternative to chocolate. It does not contain harmful ingredients such as caffeine and theobromine which are present in chocolate.

Coconut Although a saturated fat it does contain nutritional properties.
Not to be used indiscriminately.

Cornflour Can be used as a thickener. It gives a similar result to kuzu and does not produce the stringiness that arrowroot does. Although it is not desirable because it is highly refined, and some people may be sensitive to corn, it is far less expensive than kuzu and does not become rubbery like arrowroot.

Dried Fruit Very nutritious, but use sparingly as it has a high sugar content. Be sure to obtain unsulphured dried fruit since the treated variety may cause unpleasant side effects.

Eggs Nutritious but care should be taken not to eat too many, due to their high cholesterol content. Always obtain 'free range' eggs as these hens have been allowed to live naturally, have not been caged and are not fed antibiotics or hormones. Duck, quail or turkey eggs are sometimes tolerated when hen eggs are not.

Fats A high fat intake has been linked with many degenerative diseases such as some cancers and coronary artery disease, therefore a low fat diet is desirable to maintain good health.

Ghee Clarified butter. The butter has been changed by heating and skimming. This removes the proteins, water and unstable fats which cause butter to become rancid. Ghee keeps well and does not burn when heated. Use sparingly. For recipe see 'sauteeing' in Cooking Methods.

Grains Ideally as many grains as tolerated should be included in our diet, in order to obtain as many nutrients as possible. In the case of allergies, use only those that do not cause undesirable symptoms. Millet and buckwheat are particularly nutritious and are more likely to be tolerated than the other grains.

Herbs Add flavour and interest to many dishes and can be used fresh or dried. Listed below are some of the most common ones and their culinary uses.
Basil — adds flavour to tomato dishes, savoury loaves, pies and salads.
Bay leaves — can be added to soups and casseroles. Remove before serving.
Chives — have a mild onion flavour and can be added to coleslaws, cooked savoury dishes and also as a garnish.
Coriander — has a spicy aroma and is used in curries.
Cummin — is used in rice dishes and can be used alone instead of curry powder.
Dill — complements seafood.
Marjoram — adds flavour to potato and tomato dishes.
Mint — is cool and refreshing and can be used to garnish cool drinks or added to vegetable dishes or desserts.
Oregano — is useful in tomato dishes for example pizza.
Parsley — is one of the most popular herbs and can be added to any savoury dish. Use generously as a garnish. It is particularly rich in iron and vitamin C.

Rosemary — has a strong flavour, so use sparingly in stuffings or in herb scones.
Sage — is used with onions as a stuffing for fish or chicken.
Thyme — useful in rissoles, loaves and stuffings.

Hiziki   A sea vegetable, very rich in calcium and other minerals. Can be soaked and then cooked with other vegetables.

Kombu   A sea vegetable. It is mostly used in soups. It needs to be cooked for a fairly long time until soft.

Kuzu   Also known as Japanese arrowroot. It is a natural and wholesome food, and it can be used instead of cornstarch, arrowroot, flours and gelatin. Texture is smooth and not rubbery.

Lecithin   As a liquid, use in place of fats or oils for greasing cooking utensils.

Mirin   Is a naturally fermented sweet brown rice cooking wine, used to flavour vegetable dishes and desserts.

Nori   A sea vegetable. Although an unfamiliar taste at first, this may well become a favourite. A sheet of nori can be toasted under the griller until it becomes green. Use as a garnish on soups or salads or fill with cooked brown rice and make into a roll.

Nuts   Include almonds, cashews, hazelnuts, brazil nuts, pecans, pine nuts, walnuts, macadamias and pistachios. They are best eaten raw and unsalted, but can be roasted slowly in the oven or in a dry pan (no need to oil). Nuts vary in the amount of oil they contain. Almonds are regarded as the most nutritious. Peanuts are very oily, difficult to digest and are a common allergen. They are in fact a legume, not a nut. To make nut milks and nut butters, see notes on beverages and spreads.

Oils   Avoid all margarines and oils which have been treated. Use cold pressed oils in salad dressings. It is best not to cook or heat them in any way as they become rancid quickly. Keep oil intake to a minimum. Oils should be kept refrigerated.

Organic   The importance of eating organically grown food cannot be overstated. Try to obtain fresh fruit and vegetables which have been grown as free of pesticides as possible. You will notice they have a far superior flavour compared with those that are not organically grown. If it is difficult to obtain organically grown fruit and vegetables, soak your vegetables in a bowl of water to which one cup of cheap apple cider vinegar has been added. The acid solution will remove some of the poisons.

Preservatives   Enable food to last longer and look deceptively attractive. Remember that fresh food is best nutritionally and that preservatives have detrimental effects on health.

Roasting   Nuts and seeds are best eaten raw. In this way optimum nutrition is obtained. If a garnish of roasted nuts or seeds is desired, this can be done by placing them in the oven or under the griller until browned. Roasting does destroy some of the nutrients.

Seaweed   Is used extensively by the Japanese and is now becoming popular in Western countries. There are several varieties such as hiziki, wakami, kombu, and arame. They are very nutritious, rich in trace elements and iodine. The high sodium content can be greatly reduced by soaking and rinsing. It is used in pies, soups, salads and casseroles.

Seeds   An excellent source of protein and essential fatty acids. Below is a list of commonly used ones.
Sesame — unhulled variety is best. Particularly rich in calcium, even richer than cow's milk and in a more assimilative form.
Sunflower — these make a very sustaining snack and contain vitamin E and phosphorus. They are not commonly allergenic and are very versatile.
Linseed — helpful in problems with constipation as it helps lubricate the bowel.

Sprouts   A most valuable food, rich in protein, vitamins and minerals, inexpensive to prepare. See salad section for instructions.

Sweetners   There are several substitutes for sugar. Dried fruits are an alternative as are raw honey, maple syrup and rice syrup. They are high energy foods to be used with discretion.

Tahini   Made from sesame seeds ground to an oily paste. It is a highly nutritious and versatile food, useful in savoury or sweet dishes.

Tamari   A fermented soya product, similar in taste to soya sauce but lower in salt and is available in a wheat free variety.

Tea   Herb teas are an excellent substitute for the usual tea and coffee, which both have undesirable substances such as caffeine and tannin. Refreshingly delicious and therapeutically valuable, there is a great variety and combination of teas available. Some of the most common are peppermint, rosehip, camomile, alfalfa, lemon grass and linden teas.

Tofu   A soya bean curd, obtained from soya beans and made into a block form similar in appearance to cheese. It is bland flavoured, smooth textured, high in protein, low in fat and it can be sliced, cubed or blended. It combines well with savoury or sweet. We have chosen to use firm, not silken tofu.

Water   Town water supplies contain a number of harmful chemicals. Apart from chlorine and the controversial fluoride, there are many added substances some of which are carcinogenic. Therefore, it is best to use only distilled or filtered water. Filters are available at good health stores.

NOTES TO THE COOK

Practical Hints For agar to work effectively and to be smooth textured, it is best soaked in fruit juice for 1-2 hours or overnight. If soaking is not possible, it will need a longer period of heating. Should lumps remain, blend thoroughly after adding to the remaining ingredients.

Seeds and nuts are best ground for maximum assimilation, unless used as a garnish.

Every effort should be made to purchase flours as fresh as possible and they should be stored in the fridge until used. If fresh millet meal cannot be purchased, rolled millet can be ground in a good blender or Bamix to make a fine meal.

It is best to keep all grains, nuts and seeds refrigerated, especially during warm weather, to protect from nutritional loss and rancidity.

To minimise the amount of fat ingested, always remove the skin and the fat under it, prior to cooking a chicken.

Do not peel vegetables; peeling removes valuable nutrients just below the skin. It is a good idea to brush fruit and vegies with a stiff brush before using.

If you need to omit yeast from your diet add lots of fresh herbs for flavour, (dried herbs do not have the delightful flavour and aroma of fresh herbs). Parsley, chives, basil, oregano, lovage and mint are all easy to grow in your garden or in pots.

Almonds can be blanched by soaking in boiling water, the skins can then be removed easily.

Wash strawberries before removing stems as this avoids loss of juice.

When using only half an avocado leave the seed in the unused half, squeeze lemon juice over it, then cover and refrigerate. This will help to prevent browning.

Marinate tofu and keep refrigerated in a ceramic or glass container ready for a quick meal with a salad.

Save the peels from oranges and lemons, dry and chop ready for use where a recipe calls for mixed peel.

Salad dressings can be made ahead of time and kept in glass jars till needed.

Before cooking lentils, dried peas and beans, remove stones, then wash thoroughly to remove dirt.

If lemons are hard, soften by soaking in hot water.

Beetroot leaves are very nutritious and can be chopped and added to salads or used instead of spinach and silverbeet in cooking.

Bicarbonate of soda is useful for cleaning fridges, sinks, stoves and ovens.

To remove skins from tomatoes, plunge into hot water and leave for a few minutes. The skins can then be peeled off easily.

To store fresh parsley, refrigerate unwashed in an airtight jar.

Warm baking utensils before greasing as this will reduce the amount of fat required.

An alternative method to soften legumes before cooking is to bring desired quantity of water to boil. Add beans, boil one minute, turn off heat and allow to stand. Then turn on heat and simmer till tender.

Remove icecreams from fridge 10 to 15 minutes before serving, depending on weather, to allow to soften.

When thickening with potato flour, place desired amount into flour sifter and spread evenly over surface of pan.

Measurements

Note: Liquid and dry measures used in our recipes are based on the standard metric cup (1 cup = 250 ml) and the standard metric measuring spoons (1 tablespoon = 20 ml) (1 teaspoon = 5 ml).

All measurements are level unless otherwise stated.

Pie quantities are for a 20 cm dish.

Kitchen Utensils

Baking Equipment

Use stoneware, glass, ceramic, stainless steel or cast iron cooking utensils. Aluminium utensils are best avoided, due to the possibility of chemical contamination of the food. There are many harmful effects from aluminium poisoning. Although non-stick cooking utensils solve the problem of omitting fats and oils, there are some suggestions that they may be injurious to health.

Blender or Food Processor

This is a great asset for pureeing, blending, grinding and shredding and is a time saver for the busy cook.

Waffle Iron

Preferably use a cast iron waffle iron, although these are difficult to find. Use a little ghee or liquid lecithin for greasing.

Lentil and Walnut Pâté (p32) with Savoury Crackers (p116) and Seed Bread (p90)

Avocado Soup (p34) with Seed Bread (p90)

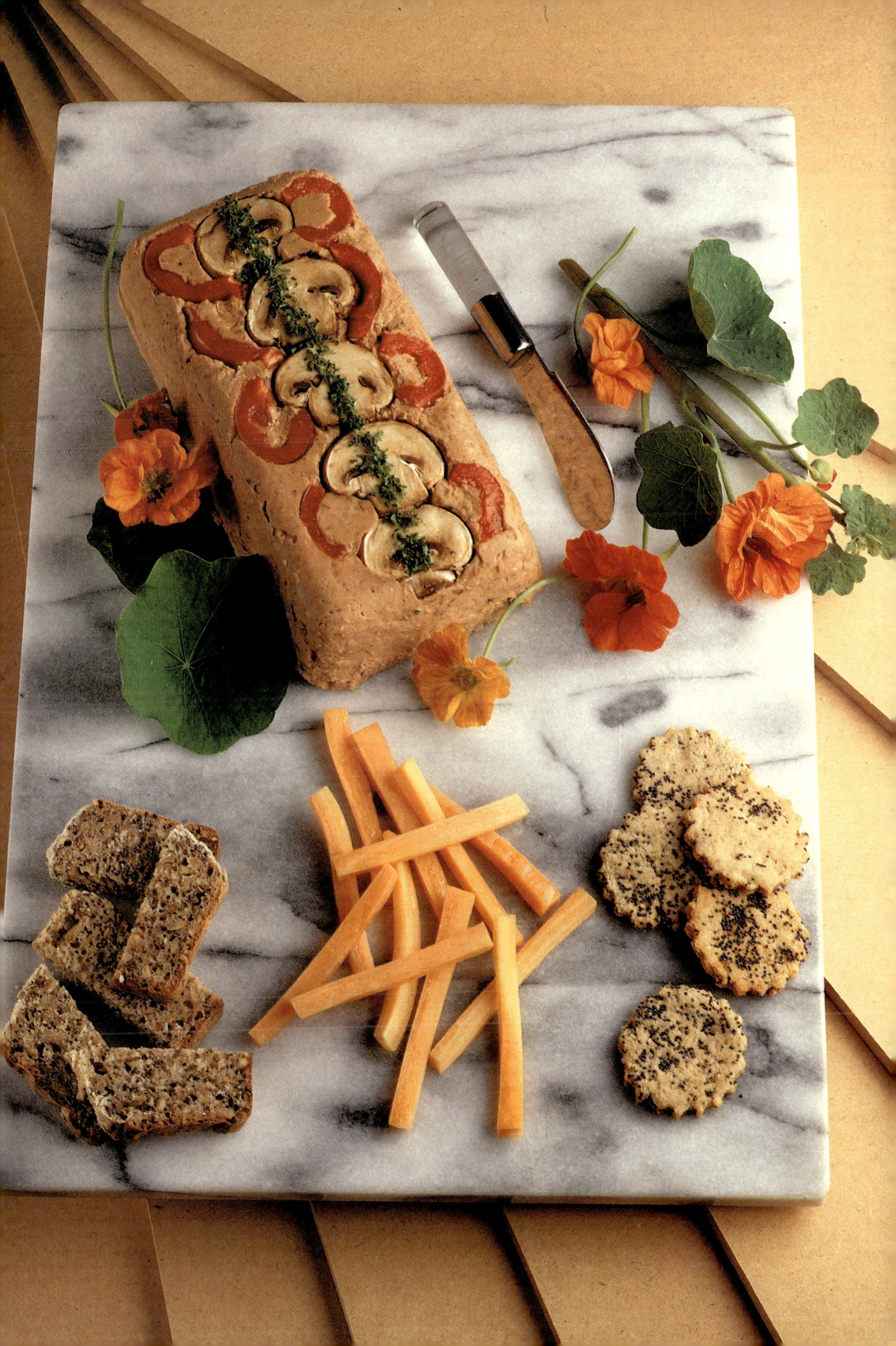

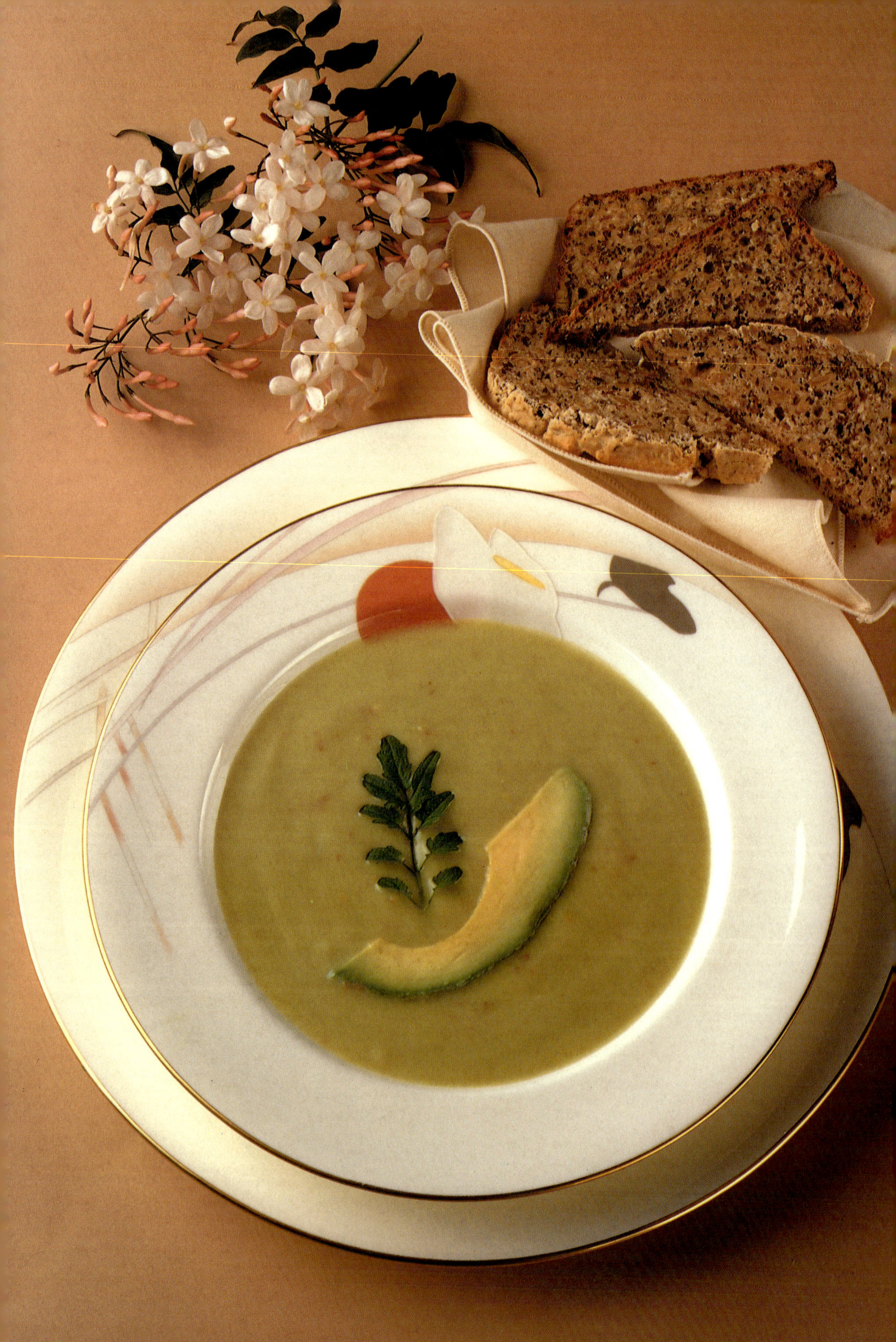

Fruit and Vegetable Juicer

Juices are best freshly made rather than bottled and tinned. They are superior in nutrition and flavour. However some bottled varieties are a convenient substitute (read labels). See the beverage section for ideas on juice combinations.

Stone Flour Mill

A good electric stone flour mill is very expensive but has the advantage of providing freshly milled grain which is not rancid, provided the mill does not heat the grain to a high temperature. Other cheaper alternatives are handmills, although these provide only small amounts of flour. Foods baked with freshly ground flour are far superior in flavour and nutrition to flours which are not fresh. However this is the ideal and it is not always possible to achieve.

Other Useful Kitchen Equipment:

brush for scrubbing vegetables
vegetable steamer
set of sharp knives
set of measuring spoons and cups
food mixer or hand beater
double saucepan
nut cracker
cropper cracker, particularly useful for macadamia nuts
muffin tin
chocolate moulds used for making carob confectionery (plastic moulds are available in a variety of shapes in delicatessens, health food shops and kitchen shops)
large bread tin (preferably made of pyrex or stoneware, not aluminium)

Cooking Methods

The cooking methods used in this book have been chosen because they require little or no fat and retain nutrients.

Steaming

Either use a vegetable steamer basket or a saucepan which requires very little water e.g. Corning Ware and stainless steel saucepans. Boiling vegetables in a lot of water results in a loss of nutrients.

Baking

When baking vegetables or chicken, place on a wire rack or tray with a little water at the bottom of the tray. There is no need to brush vegetables with oil or fat. When baking breads, cakes or biscuits, use a little liquid lecithin for greasing. Flour can be sprinkled on the bottom of the tray to prevent sticking for such things as biscuits and scones (this works well with Corning Ware).

Sauteeing

Either use a few tablespoons of water, fat free chicken stock, vegetable stock or a small amount of ghee. To make ghee, melt unsalted butter in a stainless steel, ceramic or enamel saucepan, cook on moderate heat and bring to boil, skim off froth with a wide knife or large spoon. It may be necessary to do this several times, making sure that all the white froth has been removed from the surface. Reduce heat while simmering. Flakes will appear in liquid, pour off the pure liquid when these begin to brown, leaving all sediments in bottom of saucepan. Refrigerate and use sparingly in cooking.

Poaching Food is cooked in liquid just below boiling point; fish fillets, for example, can be poached in water and lemon juice.

Crockpot Cookery A method of providing nutritious fat free meals on busy days when advance preparation is convenient; for example, breakfast prepared the night before or perhaps dinner when leaving early in the morning. Many conventional recipes can be adapted to the crockpot.

Hors d'Oeuvres

Hors d'oeuvres are small pre-dinner nibbles which need to be simple and attractively presented. They also make suitable snacks for other occasions.

Stuffed Zucchini

Free of dairy products, wheat, corn, sugar, eggs, soy and orange.
Can be yeast free if mushroom is omitted.

Makes 12

¼ cup cooked rice
1 tablespoon finely chopped tomato
1 tablespoon finely chopped capsicum
small pinch mixed herbs
1 teaspoon finely chopped shallots
1 mushroom finely chopped
1 teaspoon finely chopped onion
1 teaspoon chopped fresh basil
1-2 teaspoons tahini (to bind)
1 medium to large zucchini

Mix together rice, tomato, capsicum, herbs, shallots, mushroom, onion, basil and tahini. Cut zucchini in half lengthwise and scoop out some of the flesh, leaving a little near the skin. Fill with rice mixture. Cut into bite size pieces and serve on a bed of lettuce garnished with parsley or watercress.

Rum Prunes

Free of dairy products, wheat, corn sugar, eggs, soy and nightshades.
Can be made free of yeast by omitting rum.

prunes, as many as desired
rum or equal parts rum and orange juice or
orange juice with grated orange rind
toasted almonds (the same number as
   there are prunes)

Soak required number of prunes for several hours or overnight in liquid. Roast the almonds in moderate oven, for approximately 10 minutes or toast under griller (being careful not to burn). Remove stone from each prune and replace with an almond.

Variation:

Fill prunes with cottage cheese mixed with a little grated lemon or orange rind.

Nibble Mix

Free of dairy products, wheat, yeast, corn, sugar, eggs, soy, orange and nightshades.

A nibble mix may consist of raw or home roasted nuts and/or seeds for
example almonds, hazelnuts, cashews, pecans, sunflower seeds and
pumpkin seeds.

Nori Rolls

Free of dairy products, wheat, corn, sugar, eggs, soy and orange.
Can be made free from nightshade by omitting capsicum.

Makes 14

½ cup short grain brown rice
1 cup water
1 teaspoon cummin
juice ½ lemon
1 tablespoon apple cider vinegar
1 tablespoon each chopped chives and
    parsley
2 teaspoons tahini if necessary
strips of carrot or red capsicum
2 sheets nori seaweed

Cook rice in water till soft and sticky. Mix in
cummin, lemon juice, apple cider vinegar, chives and
parsley. (If mixture is still not holding together well
enough mix in tahini.) Toast nori under griller, one
sheet at a time until it turns green — but be careful
not to burn it. (If you are using pre-toasted nori
sheets, omit this step.) Spread half of the rice mixture
on 1 sheet of nori lengthwise, leaving approximately
4 cm clear along far edge. Lay strips of carrot or
capsicum lengthwise on rice mixture, so that when
the nori sheet is rolled and sliced the carrot or
capsicum will be in the middle. Dip fingers in water
and roll nori into a log shape, sealing the ends and
edges, this can take a bit of practice. Starting at one
end, cut nori into 2 cm slices using a sharp knife.
Garnish with sprigs of parsley.

Crudites with dips

Crudites are simply raw vegetables served as an appetiser. Allow a
selection of raw vegetables for each person e.g. 2 carrot sticks, 2 celery
sticks, 2 zucchini sticks, 2 strips red capsicum and 2 small
cauliflowerettes. Green beans, snow peas, broccoli, radishes and other
vegetables may also be included. Offer a choice of 2 dips or sauces such
as avocado dip, hummus, curried tofu, or yoghurt dressing. Crudités are
easy for the busy hostess to prepare.

Hummus

Free of dairy products, wheat, yeast, corn, sugar, eggs, soy, orange and nightshades.

1 cup cooked chick peas ¼ cup vegetable stock or water ⅓ cup tahini ¼ cup lemon juice 1 clove crushed garlic a little finely chopped parsley and basil pinch sea salt (optional)	Blend all ingredients together thoroughly except parsley and basil. Mix in herbs. Garnish with whole cooked chick peas or slices of lemon, dusted with paprika.

Avocado Dip

Free of dairy products, wheat, yeast, corn, sugar, eggs, soy and orange.

2-3 ripe mashed avocados 1 finely chopped tomato a little finely chopped celery and onion pinch chilli powder (optional) juice 1 lemon	Combine all ingredients.

Curried Tofu Dip

Free of dairy products, wheat, corn sugar, eggs and orange.

1 cup mashed tofu juice 1 lemon ½ teaspoon cummin 1-2 cloves crushed garlic 1 teaspoon curry powder 1 teaspoon honey or rice syrup (optional) dash tamari or sea salt (optional)	Blend all ingredients. Garnish with sprig of parsley or chopped shallots.

Potato Straws

Free of dairy products, wheat, yeast, corn, sugar, eggs, soy and orange.

500 g potatoes, or as much as required	Wash potatoes. Cut into matchstick straws. Place straws on a lightly greased tray and bake in moderate oven approximately 1 hour, or until browned and crunchy. Nice to nibble on!

Curried Eggs
Free of wheat, corn, sugar, soy, orange.

---

6 medium to large eggs (hard boiled and
   shelled)

2 teaspoons non fat yoghurt or to
   consistency desired

1 teaspoon honey

1-2 teaspoons curry powder (to taste)

1 teaspoon cummin

Variation
**Free of dairy products, wheat, corn, sugar,
orange.**

¾ cup mashed tofu

1 teaspoon lemon juice

1 teaspoon curry powder

1 teaspoon cummin

1 teaspoon honey

dash herbal seasoning (optional)

Slice eggs lengthwise and carefully remove yolks. Combine mashed yolks, yoghurt, honey, curry powder and cummin. Mix until smooth and creamy. With a small spoon place mixture into egg whites. Dust with paprika.

Combine ingredients and place into egg whites.

Savoury Crackers

Suitable rice crackers, or see savoury
   biscuits in biscuit section

Spreads such as cottage cheese, nut
   butters, avocado, hummus, lentil and
   walnut pâté (see other sections)

Garnishes such as parsley, nasturtiums,
   watercress, radishes and carrot curls

Spread crackers with any of the above suggestions. Add garnishes for colour and interest (see below).

Carrot Curls
Free of dairy products, wheat, yeast, corn, sugar, eggs, soy, orange and nightshades.

Peel carrot lengthwise with potato peeler to obtain several long thin
strips. Curl around a pencil or finger. Secure with a toothpick. Place in
ice cold water until curls hold their shape when toothpick is removed.

Fish Cocktail Pieces

Free of dairy products, wheat, corn, sugar, eggs, soy and orange.
Free of nightshades and yeast if sauce is not used.

Makes 48

500 g fish
½-¾ cup allowable flour
½-¾ cup nut or soy milk
1 ½ cups lightly toasted sesame seeds or
ground almonds
1 quantity sweet and sour sauce (optional)
see Sauce section

Cut fresh fish into bite size pieces, removing any bones. Roll in flour, then in nut or soy milk, finally roll in toasted sesame seeds or almonds. Spread fish pieces onto a lightly greased tray. Bake in moderate oven approximately 30 minutes.

Serve fish with cocktail forks and a dish of sauce for dipping.

ENTREES

An entree is an introduction to a fine meal. Ideally it is small and is designed to stimulate rather than satisfy the appetite.

Avocado Vinaigrette

Free of dairy products, wheat, yeast, corn, sugar, eggs, soy, orange.
Free of nightshades if capsicum is not used.

Serves 4

2 medium ripe avocados
4 lettuce leaves
chopped parsley, chives or thinly sliced
   red capsicum

Cut avocados in half lengthwise and remove stones. Place each avocado half on a lettuce leaf. Pour a French dressing over avocados and then garnish.

Minted Pineapple

Free dairy products, wheat, yeast, corn, sugar, eggs, soy, orange and nightshades.

Serves 4

2 small fresh pineapples
¼ cup chopped fresh mint leaves
1 fresh cherry or strawberry per serving

Slice pineapples in half lengthwise, leaving leaves attached. Scoop out pineapple flesh and chop into bite-size pieces. Mix together pineapple and mint and replace in shells. Decorate each serving with a cherry or strawberry.

Steamed Asparagus

Free of dairy products, wheat, corn, sugar, eggs, orange and nightshades.
Can be free of soy if coconut white sauce is used.

Serves 4

20 tender asparagus spears
a little water
3 tablespoons apple cider vinegar
1 quantity Nugget sauce or white sauce
   (see recipes in Sauce section)
finely chopped parsley or basil

Steam asparagus in the water and vinegar. Serve covered with sauce. Garnish with parsley or basil.

Salad Kebabs

These are another attractive way of serving raw vegetables as an
appetiser. Skewer a variety of vegetables such as button mushrooms,
cherry tomatoes, chunks of capsicum, celery, chopped snow peas,
radishes, and serve with a sauce or dressing on a bed of sprouts or
shredded lettuce.

Stuffed Mushrooms

Free of dairy products, wheat, corn, sugar, eggs, soy and orange.   *Serves 4-6*

1 cup mashed potato
½ cup ground almonds
1 tablespoon finely chopped onion
dash tamari or herbal seasoning (optional)
1 tablespoon finely chopped celery
1 tablespoon finely chopped parsley
1 tablespoon finely chopped capsicum
2 teaspoons chopped chives
1 teaspoon chopped fresh basil
½-1 teaspoon curry powder
1 teaspoon ground cummin
16 medium-large mushrooms

Mix together all ingredients except mushrooms. Wipe
mushrooms with a damp cloth and cut off caps. Fill
mushrooms with potato mixture. Bake for 15 minutes
on a lightly greased tray in a moderate oven. Place
under griller for a few minutes so that top of mixture
is crunchy.

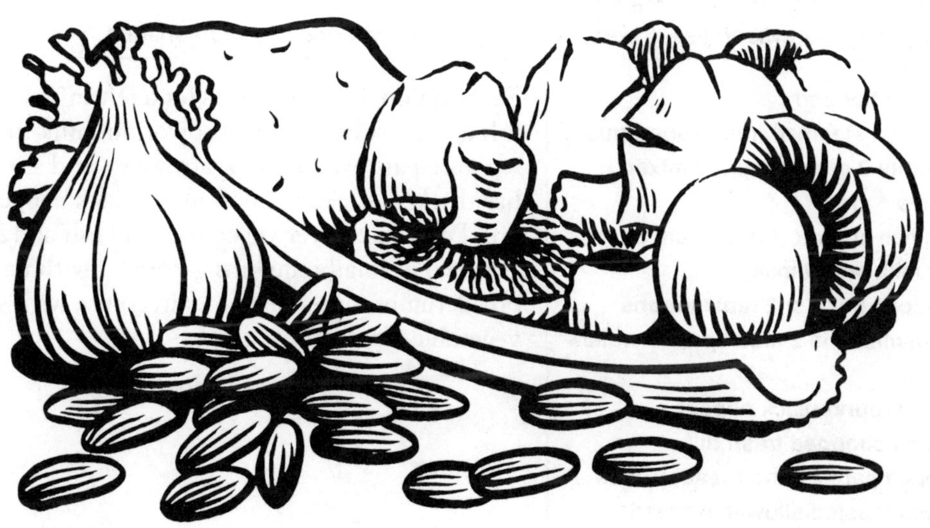

Lentil and Walnut Pâté

Free of dairy products, wheat, corn, sugar, eggs, soy and orange.
For a yeast-free pâté, omit mushrooms, tamari and mirin.

Serves 8

2 tablespoons agar* flakes

1 cup tomato puree (made by blending
   3 small tomatoes)

¼ cup vegetable stock or carrot juice

1 medium onion, chopped finely

2 cloves crushed garlic

¼ cup chopped mushrooms

1 cup cooked brown lentils (refer to note
   below recipe)

1 cup walnuts, well ground to a paste

1 cup steamed and mashed carrots
   (approximately 250 g raw)

¼ teaspoon ground oregano

1 tablespoon tomato paste

1 tablespoon chopped fresh basil

1 tablespoon tamari (optional)

2 tablespoons mirin or sherry

Soak agar flakes in tomato puree and stock or carrot juice for 1-2 hours. Saute onion, garlic and mushrooms. Combine or blend onion, garlic, mushrooms, lentils, walnuts, carrots, oregano, tomato paste, basil, tamari and mirin or sherry. Bring agar mixture to the boil, then simmer till agar flakes have dissolved. Stir agar mixture into lentil mixture, mixing well. Spoon into loaf tin (no need to grease tin). Either refrigerate till set, or bake for 20-30 minutes in a moderate oven and then chill. When set, run a knife around edges of pate and invert onto a plate. Decorate with walnut halves, thinly sliced mushrooms or sprigs of herbs.

Serve with crackers.

Note: ½ cup raw brown lentils when cooked makes approximately 1 cup. To cook lentils, wash well, place in pan and cover with water. Bring to boil, then simmer 20-30 minutes till soft. Drain off water.

* See note on agar in glossary.

Savoury Fish and Vegetables

Free of dairy products, wheat, yeast, corn, sugar, eggs, soy, orange and nightshades.

Serves 4-6

1 large onion, chopped

2 cups chopped steamed fresh asparagus
   or substitute 2 cups chopped mixed
   vegetables

400 g fresh fish cut into 1 and ½ cm cubes

2 cups soy milk or nut milk

2-3 tablespoons kuzu or 2 tablespoons
   arrowroot mixed in 2 tablespoons water

juice 1 lemon

dash freshly ground black pepper

2 tablespoons chopped fresh dill

finely chopped parsley and breadcrumbs
   made from toasted allowable bread

Saute onion and vegetables for a few minutes. Add fish and cook briefly. Heat soy or nut milk in a separate pan. Add kuzu or arrowroot and stir till milk has thickened. Add lemon juice, black pepper and dill. Pour sauce over vegetables and fish and mix well.

Serve in small ramekins garnished with parsley and breadcrumbs, or serve as a main course with steamed vegetables or salad.

Pineapple and Fish Tartlets

Free of dairy products, wheat, corn, sugar, eggs, soy, orange and nightshades.
Serves 8

Base

1 quantity pizza base, rolled and cut into rounds to fit into small patty tins, greased lightly

Filling

125 g boneless fish fillets (e.g. ocean perch) steamed and flaked
½-¾ cup cooked brown rice
½ cup chopped fresh pineapple
2 tablespoons chopped and toasted cashews or almonds
½ cup pineapple sauce

Pineapple Sauce

¾ cup unsweetened pineapple juice
1 teaspoon apple cider vinegar
¼-½ teaspoon fine grated ginger
1 tablespoon chopped chives
1 tablespoon arrowroot mixed in 1 tablespoon water

Lightly bake bases for 5-10 minutes. Combine all ingredients for filling in a bowl, except sauce. Spoon filling into pastry cases. Heat ingredients for sauce in a pan and stir till thickened. Pour over 1-2 teaspoons of sauce, just enough to flavour and combine ingredients. Bake in a moderate oven for 10 minutes until heated through.

Serve with a parsley and cress garnish.

SOUPS

Soups are easy to prepare and can make a hearty meal in themselves. They can be varied simply by using a wide range of vegetables in season, and by pureeing all or half of the soup. Suitable garnishes include finely chopped herbs, crumbled toasted nori sea vegetable or sprouts.

Soup Stock

Vegetable stock is easy to prepare by simmering a variety of vegetables in water for half an hour, then allowing to stand for a further 30 minutes. Suitable vegetables are onions, garlic, potatoes, green leafy vegetables including beet and celery tops, zucchini, pea pods, shallot tips, lettuce, beans, parsnip and parsley stems. Small quantities of defatted chicken stock may be added for flavour if desired.

Simple and delicious soups can be easily prepared by simmering a choice of vegetables in water till tender and then blending e.g. spinach, kumara and onion is an excellent combination.

Avocado Soup

Free of dairy products, wheat, corn, sugar, eggs and orange.
Free of yeast and soy if tamari is omitted.

Serves 8

6 cups water or stock
2 large onions, chopped
2 medium potatoes, grated
1 cup soy milk or nut milk
2 avocados, mashed
7 ½ cm strip lemon rind
2 tablespoons lemon juice
2 tablespoons tamari or dash herbal
    seasoning (optional)
sprinkle black pepper
dash tabasco (optional)

Place water, onions and potatoes in pan. Bring to boil and simmer 10 minutes or till potatoes and onions are soft. Add soy or nut milk, avocados, lemon rind and lemon juice. Blend till smooth and return to hotplate. Add tamari, black pepper and tabasco. Serve garnished with chopped chives or parsley. Can be served chilled if desired.

Easy Pumpkin Soup

Free of dairy products, wheat, yeast, corn, sugar, eggs, soy, orange and nightshades.   *Serves 4-5*

1 kg peeled and cut pumpkin
1 chopped onion or ½ leek, washed
3 cups vegetable stock or water
¼ cup chopped parsley
1 tablespoon finely chopped fresh basil
pinch sea salt (optional)

Place pumpkin and onion in saucepan with stock or water and simmer till pumpkin is soft. Blend till smooth and return to hotplate. Add herbs and sea salt.

Sundowner Soup

Free of dairy products, wheat, yeast, corn, sugar, eggs, soy and orange.   *Serves 6*

1 litre vegetable stock or water
2 finely chopped celery stalks
1 finely chopped onion
1-2 grated carrots
1 grated parsnip
¾ cup diced potato
¼ cup chopped parsley
1 tablespoon tomato paste
1-2 bay leaves
1 teaspoon finely chopped fresh basil
1 clove garlic, crushed
¼ teaspoon fresh ginger, grated

Place all ingredients in pan. Bring to the boil and simmer gently for about half an hour. Remove bay leaves and blend soup if a smoother texture is required.

Borscht

Free of dairy products, wheat, yeast, corn, sugar, eggs, soy, orange and nightshades.   *Serves 6*

2 large beetroots, peeled and chopped
1 onion, chopped
1 cup chopped carrot
3 cups finely chopped red cabbage
1 litre vegetable stock, or a mixture of
    vegetable and chicken stock
2 tablespoons lemon juice
2 tablespoons finely chopped parsley
2 tablespoons finely chopped fresh dill
freshly ground black pepper
pinch sea salt (optional)

Bring first five ingredients to the boil, then simmer till vegetables are tender. Blend all or half of the soup. Return to stove, add remaining ingredients and reheat.

Winter Lentil Soup

Free dairy products, wheat, yeast, corn, sugar, eggs, soy and orange. *Serves 6-8*

½ cup brown lentils, washed
1 medium carrot, grated
1 small parsnip, grated
1 small swede, grated
1 tablespoon grated ginger
1 zucchini, grated
1 medium potato, diced
1 onion, chopped
1 litre vegetable stock or water
1 cup mashed pumpkin
¼ cup chopped parsley

Place all ingredients except parsley, in a large saucepan. Bring to boil, then simmer about 40 minutes. Just before serving, stir in parsley.

Chick Pea Soup

Free of dairy products, wheat, yeast, corn, sugar, eggs, soy, orange and nightshades. *Serves 6-8*

¾ cup chick peas
1 cup chopped onion
2 cloves crushed garlic
1 cup chopped celery
¾ cup sliced green beans
2 cups chopped sweet potato
1 chopped medium zucchini
1 litre vegetable stock or water
1 teaspoon dried basil
pinch cinnamon
2 teaspoons finely chopped fresh ginger
1 bay leaf
1-2 cups mashed steamed pumpkin

Soak chick peas overnight or for 3 hours. Discard water, cover chick peas with fresh water and simmer till soft (1-2 hours). Drain and set aside. Saute onion, garlic, celery, beans, sweet potato and zucchini. Cover vegetables with stock or water. Add turmeric, basil, cinnamon, ginger and bay leaf. Simmer until the vegetables are tender. Add the cooked chick peas and pumpkin and remove bay leaf.

Pea Soup

Free of dairy products, wheat, yeast, corn, sugar, eggs, soy, orange and nightshades. *Serves 4-6*

1 cup dried yellow or green split peas
5 cups water
2 pieces kombu sea vegetable
1 large onion, chopped
½ cup chopped celery
½ cup chopped celery leaves
½ cup chopped carrot
½ cup chopped parsley
2 tablespoons chopped mint

Wash peas well. Bring peas to boil in water and simmer for half an hour. Add kombu and simmer together with peas for a further half an hour or until soft. Add remaining ingredients and simmer till tender. Garnish with chopped mint.

Pumpkin Soup

Free of dairy products, wheat, yeast, corn, sugar, eggs, soy, orange and can be free of nightshades if alternatives are used.
Serves 6-8

1 whole pumpkin, approximately 5 kg
1 large onion, chopped
1 large parsnip or potato, peeled and
   chopped
1 litre vegetable stock, or a mixture of
   vegetable and chicken stock
1 kg chopped pumpkin (see step 4)
½ cup tomato juice or ½ cup carrot or
   celery juice plus juice ½ lemon
extra stock to thin soup if necessary
pinch nutmeg
pinch sea salt (optional)
2 tablespoons finely chopped fresh basil
2 tablespoons finely chopped fresh chives
   or parsley

This makes an impressive and inexpensive entree for a winter dinner party.

Place whole pumpkin upside down in baking dish containing approximately 3 cm water. Cover baking dish with foil and bake pumpkin about 1 hour in moderate oven. Remove from oven. Turn pumpkin right way up and cut a circle from the top, leaving a 2 cm rim around the edge of the pumpkin. Scoop out the flesh and seeds, using a sharp knife and leaving a 2 cm wall. Reserve 1 kg flesh for the soup. Place pumpkin, onion, parsnip or potato and stock in saucepan, bring to boil, then simmer about 20 minutes. Blend soup, then return to stove. Add tomato juice or carrot or celery juice with lemon. Add extra stock if necessary. Season to taste with nutmeg and sea salt. Reheat gently.

Place pumpkin onto a suitable plate and decorate with ivy. Pour soup into pumpkin shell and stir in basil. Garnish with parsley or chives. Serve with savoury biscuits (see Biscuit section) or toasted seed bread.

Leek and Broccoli Soup

Free of dairy products, wheat, yeast, corn, sugar, eggs, soy, orange and nightshades.
Serves 6-8

5 cups stock — chicken, vegetable or a
   mixture
750 g chopped broccoli
2 medium leeks
1 chopped onion
Herbal seasoning or sea salt or tamari to
   taste
dash freshly ground black pepper if
desired

Place stock, broccoli, leeks and onion in a saucepan, bring to the boil, then simmer till vegetables are tender. Blend thoroughly. Reheat slowly and add seasonings.

Serve garnished with finely chopped parsley or chives.

SALADS

With their great variety of tastes, textures and colours, salads provide some of the most attractive and delicious dishes for the table. Containing an abundance of vitamins, minerals and enzymes, raw vegetables are highly nutritious and a large salad with lunch or dinner every day is an enormous contribution toward good health.

Exciting and creative salads are merely a matter of combining a variety of complementary vegetables and a suitable dressing.

Sprouts

Any seeds for example alfalfa, fenugreek, mustard, radish, sesame, sunflower, aduki beans, chick peas, mung beans, soya beans, unhulled millet
jar, for soaking seeds
gauze or mesh
elastic band

Place a quantity of seeds into a jar, approximately ½ cup, depending on size of jar. Rinse seeds well then cover with plenty of water. Leave to soak overnight. Drain water from seeds, rinse and drain once more. Place in warm spot. Every day rinse and drain until sprouts shoot. This can take anything from 2-5 days, depending on type of sprout and warmth of weather. After about three days place seeds in the sun for a few hours to develop the chlorophyll. Store in a jar in fridge and use on salads or with vegetables.

Sprout Salad

Free of dairy products, wheat, corn, sugar, eggs, soy and nightshades.
Can be made free of yeast by omitting raisins.
Can be made free of orange juice.

2 cups any sprouts singly or combined, for example: mung, alfalfa, lentil, red clover and/or fenugreek
¼ cup parsley finely chopped
2 tablespoons finely chopped raisins or fresh dates
2 tablespoons pumpkin seeds
lemon or orange juice

Mix together sprouts, parsley, raisins or dates and pumpkin seeds. Squeeze a little lemon or orange juice over salad.

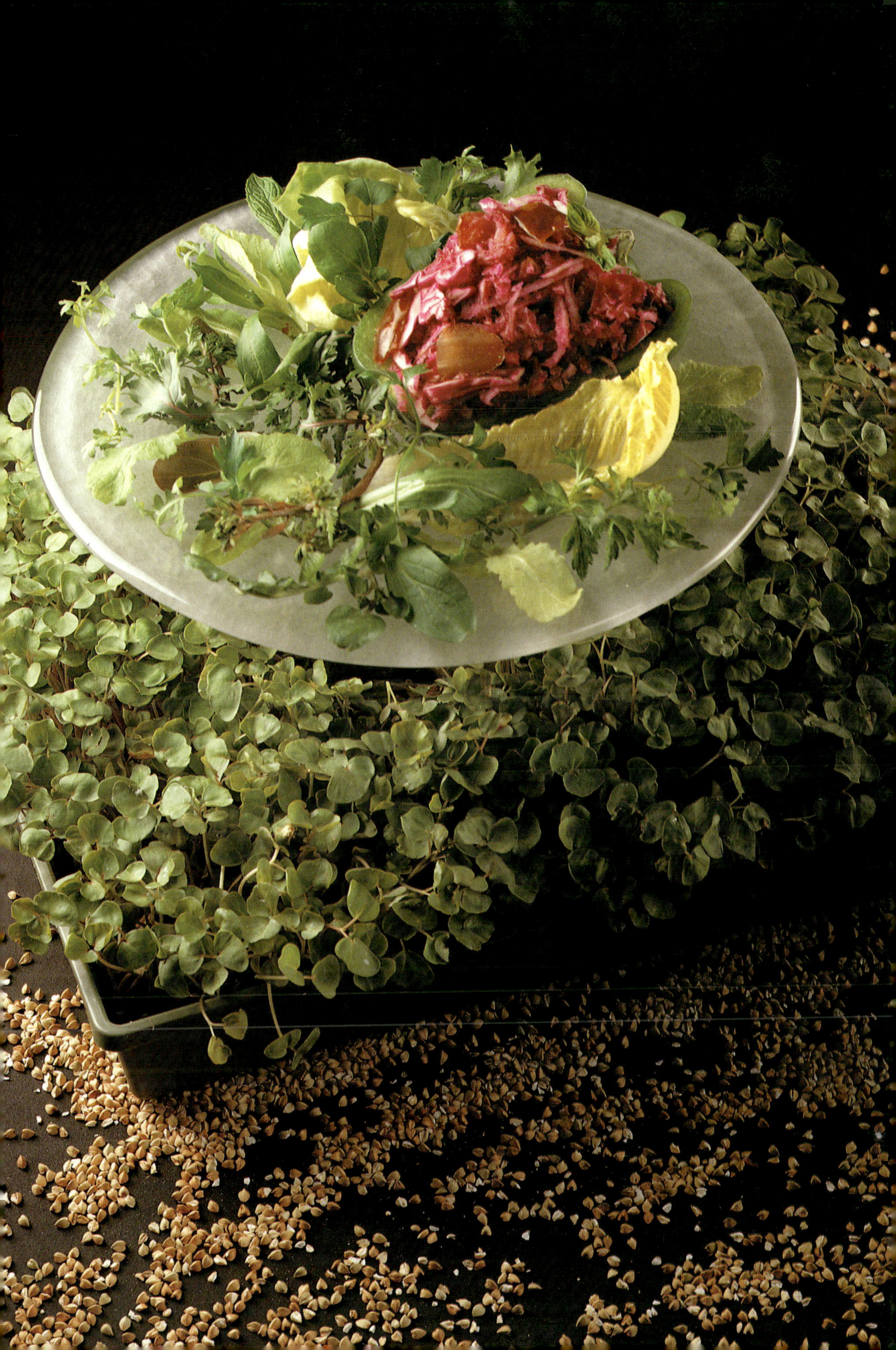

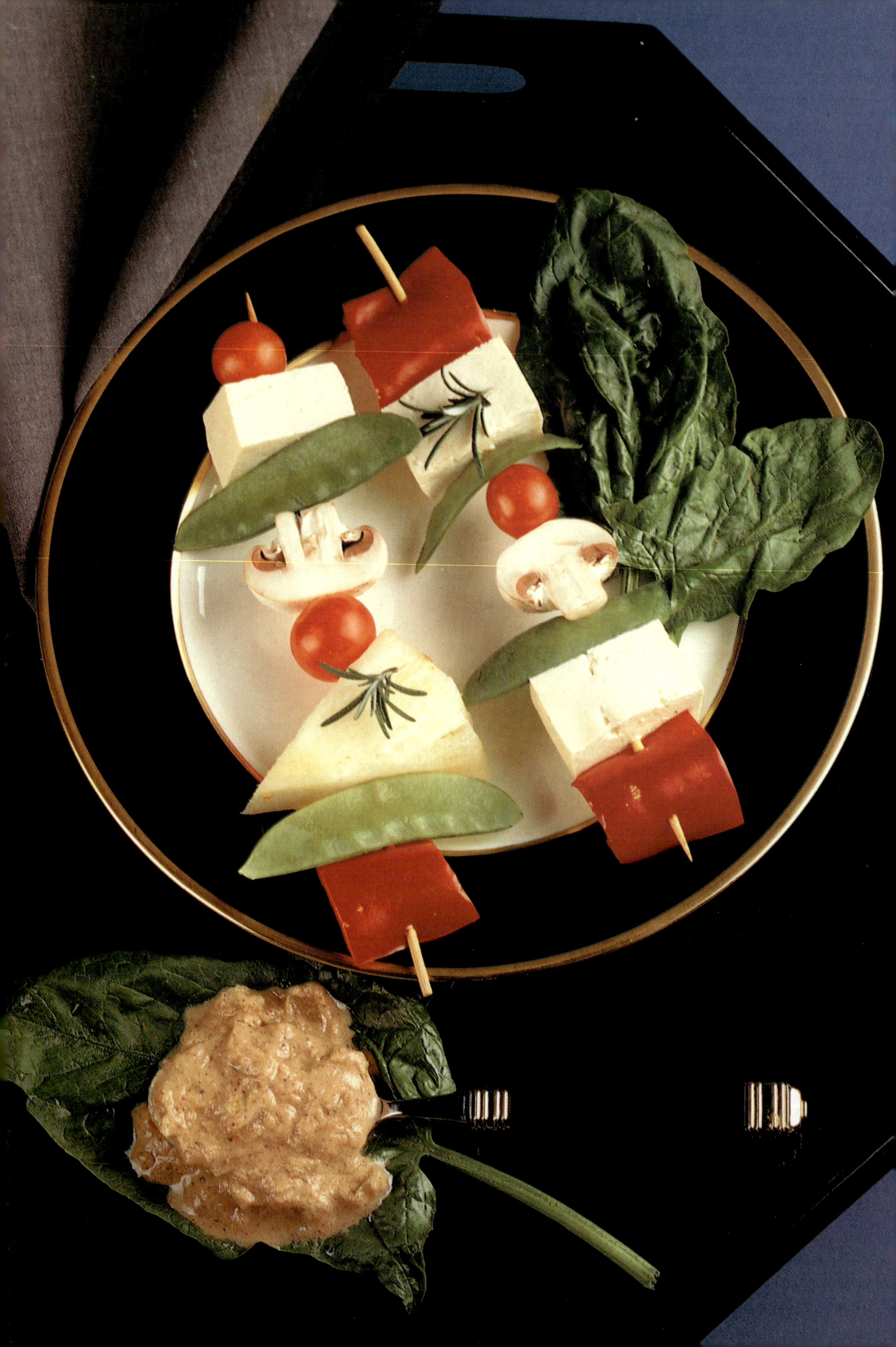

Tomato and Cucumber Salad

Free of dairy products, wheat, corn, sugar, eggs, soy and orange.

¾ **cup spring onions (cut into rings)** ¼ **cup apple cider vinegar** 1 **cup sliced tomato** 1 **cup sliced cucumber** 1-2 **tablespoons finely chopped fresh basil**	Mix together onion and vinegar and leave to stand 1-2 hours. Drain off vinegar if desired. Add tomato, cucumber and basil, mix well.

Coleslaw

Free of dairy products, wheat, yeast, corn, sugar, eggs, soy and orange.

3 **cups finely chopped cabbage** ¾ **cup finely chopped celery** ¼ **cup finely chopped red capsicum** 1 **cup grated carrot** ¾ **cup finely chopped pineapple, apple or** **grapes** ¼ **cup pineapple or apple juice**	Combine ingredients, mixing thoroughly. Coleslaw may be varied by using grated pumpkin, grated cucumber or corn kernels.

Carrot and Raisin Salad

Free of dairy, wheat, corn, sugar, eggs, soy and nightshades.
Can be made free of yeast by omitting raisins.

2 **cups grated carrot** ¼ **cup desiccated coconut** 2 **tablespoons finely chopped raisins or** **fresh dates** **juice** ½ **orange**	Mix ingredients well together.

Green Salad

Free of dairy products, wheat, yeast, corn, sugar, eggs, soy and orange.
Can be made free of nightshades by omitting capsicums.

Use any of the following: buckwheat and
    sunflower, lettuce, cabbage, celery,
    capsicum, shallots, green beans,
    zucchini, cucumber, sprouts, dandelion
    leaves, endive, spinach and parsley.
    Different lettuces can be used, for
    example mignonette, iceberg and cos.
	Wash and dry vegetables. Chop or tear. Toss together in a bowl and serve with dressing of choice (see Dressings section).
	    A green salad can have many variations, depending on whatever vegetables are in season.

Buckwheat Lettuce (p43) capsicum filled with Purple Salad (p46) buckwheat groats

Tofu Kebabs (p40) with Spicy Nut Sauce (p88)

Tabouli Salad

Free of dairy products, wheat, yeast, corn, sugar, eggs, soy and orange.

⅓ **cup toasted sunflower or sesame seeds (or a mixture of both)** **2 cups finely chopped parsley** ¼ **cup finely chopped shallots** ¼ **cup finely chopped mint** **juice 1 lemon** **1 finely chopped tomato**	Mix all ingredients. **Variation:** Substitute seeds with 1 cup cooked brown rice or ⅓ cup raw buckwheat which has been soaked in water for 1 hour and then drained.

Avocado Salad

Free of dairy products, wheat, yeast, corn, sugar, eggs, soy, orange and nightshades.

1 avocado (sliced) **lettuce leaves** **alfalfa sprouts** **dressing of choice**	Arrange sliced avocado on lettuce leaves and top with alfalfa sprouts. Cover with dressing of choice.

Purple Salad

Free of dairy products, wheat, corn, sugar, eggs, soy, orange and nightshades.
Can be made free of yeast if fresh dates are used and apple cider vinegar is omitted.

3 cups finely shredded red cabbage ¼ **cup chopped dates** **1 large carrot or apple, grated** **2 cloves crushed garlic** **finely chopped ginger to taste, as much as liked** ¼ **cup apple juice or a mixture of apple juice and apple cider vinegar**	Mix all ingredients well together.

Waldorf Salad

Free of wheat, corn, sugar, eggs, soy, orange and nightshades.
Can be made free of dairy products, and yeast if lemon juice is substituted for yoghurt.

2 cups diced unpeeled apple **1 cup chopped celery** ½ **cup chopped walnuts or pecans** **2 tablespoons non fat yoghurt or juice of half a lemon (optional)**	Mix all ingredients well together.

Orange and Avocado Salad

Free of dairy products, wheat, yeast, corn, sugar, eggs, soy and nightshades.

2 avocados (skins and stones removed)
1-2 oranges (peeled and chopped)
1 spring onion or small onion, cut into rings
2 tablespoons lemon juice
2 tablespoons orange juice
¼ teaspoon oil (optional)
¼ teaspoon chopped fresh ginger
lettuce leaves

Cut avocados into slices lengthwise. Mix with orange pieces and onion rings. Mix together lemon juice, orange juice, oil and ginger, then pour over salad.

Serve on lettuce leaves.

Beetroot Salad

Free of dairy products, wheat, yeast, corn, sugar, eggs, soy, orange and nightshades.

1 large beetroot (grated)
juice 1 lemon

Mix beetroot and lemon juice together.

Variation:

Add 1 grated apple and 1 teaspoon finely chopped fresh ginger.

Sweet Potato Salad

Free of dairy products, wheat, yeast, corn, sugar, eggs, soy, orange and nightshades.

600 g kumera
1 tablespoon cold pressed oil or apple juice
3 tablespoons lemon juice
1-2 cloves crushed garlic
1 tablespoon chopped parsley
1 tablespoon chopped basil
1 tablespoon chopped chives
1 tablespoon chopped spring onion

Steam kumera till tender but not mushy. Dice and place in a bowl. Add remaining ingredients and stir well.

Serve with salad vegetables.

Gherkins

Free of dairy products, wheat, corn, sugar, eggs, soy, orange and nightshades.

6 fresh gherkins, washed thoroughly
¾ cup water
pinch sea salt
¼ cup apple cider vinegar
1 tablespoon lemon juice
1 tablespoon honey

Cook gherkins in water and salt till tender but not mushy. Add remaining ingredients. Pour into a jar and refrigerate.

Rice Salad

Free of dairy products, wheat, corn, sugar, eggs, soy and orange.
Can be made free of yeast by using French Dressing No 2.

3 cups cooked rice
¾ cup cooked peas
¼ cup finely chopped red capsicum
2 tablespoons finely chopped parsley
2 tablespoons finely chopped shallots or
** chives**
¼ cup French dressing (see Dressing
** section)**
½ teaspoon ground turmeric
1 teaspoon ground cummin
2 tablespoons toasted sesame seeds

Mix together rice, peas, capsicum, parsley and shallots. Add turmeric and cummin to dressing and pour over rice mixture, mixing well. Stir in sesame seeds and serve.

Chicken and Rice Salad

Free of wheat, corn, sugar, eggs, soy and nightshades.
Can be made free of dairy products by omitting yoghurt.
Can be made free of yeast by using Olive Mayonnaise.

1 cup cooked rice
1 cup cooked chicken
1 cup chopped shallots
¼ cup chopped celery
1 tablespoon chopped parsley
1 tablespoon non fat yoghurt or Tahini
** Mayonnaise or Olive Mayonnaise**
2 tablespoons orange rind, finely grated
¼ cup almonds (skins removed and
browned lightly under griller)

Combine all ingredients except mayonnaise, orange rind and almonds. Stir through mayonnaise and orange rind. Serve on lettuce leaves and top with almonds.

Buckwheat Lettuce

**1 cup buckwheat sprouting seeds
   (unhulled buckwheat)**
2 seed trays (approximately 28 x 33 cm)
peat moss
soil or compost soil

Soak buckwheat seeds in water to cover, for 12 hours or overnight. Drain off water. Spread peat over tray approximately 2 cm in depth. Spread soil over peat, also approximately 2 cm deep. Spread seeds evenly over the soil. Place a damp tea towel over seeds and leave for 2-3 days. Keep tea towel damp. Remove tea towel. Keep seeds moist but do not overwater. Buckwheat lettuce will be ready to cut after a week or slightly longer. Add to salads for variety and flavour.

Sunflower Lettuce

Follow method for buckwheat lettuce, using sunflower sprouting seeds (unhulled sunflower seeds), which are available from some well stocked health food stores. Sunflower lettuce also makes a tasty addition to salads.

Buckwheat and sunflower lettuces are very economical especially when other green vegetables are expensive. Like sprouts they have the advantage of being home grown, organic and fresh from the garden.

DRESSINGS

Fresh vegetables have a taste and flavour all their own. A good dressing should complement these natural flavours and should never overpower them.

French Dressing (1)

Free of dairy products, wheat, corn, sugar, eggs, soy, orange and nightshades.

1-2 tablespoons cold-pressed oil **¼ cup lemon juice** **3 tablespoons apple cider vinegar** **1 clove crushed garlic** **dash lemon pepper** **1 tablespoon finely chopped herbs** **e.g. parsley, chives, basil** **1 teaspoon honey**	Blend ingredients, or shake together in a jar.

French Dressing (2)

Free of dairy products, wheat, yeast, corn, sugar, eggs, soy, orange and nightshades.

¾ cup fresh apple juice **¼ cup lemon juice** **1 clove garlic, crushed** **1 tablespoon finely chopped fresh herbs** **e.g. parsley, chives, basil**	Combine ingredients.

Yoghurt Dressing

Free of wheat, corn, sugar, eggs, soy, orange and nightshades.

½ cup goat's yoghurt or non-fat yoghurt **1 tablespoon lemon or orange juice** **1 teaspoon finely chopped fresh basil** **or dill** **1 clove crushed garlic**	Combine ingredients.

Tofu Dressing

Free of dairy products, wheat, corn, sugar, eggs, orange and nightshades.

1 cup mashed tofu 2 tablespoons lemon juice 3 tablespoons tahini 1 teaspoon tamari 1 tablespoon finely chopped spring onion 1 tablespoon finely chopped chives 1 tablespoon finely chopped parsley	Blend tofu, lemon juice, tahini and tamari. Stir in onion, chives and parsley.

Avocado Dressing

Free of dairy products, wheat, yeast, corn, sugar, eggs, soy and orange.

1 large avocado
1 large tomato
1 spring onion, chopped
2 teaspoons chopped fresh dill or
   1 teaspoon dried dill
1 teaspoon chopped fresh oregano or
   ½ teaspoon dried oregano
	Blend ingredients and serve over sprouts, cooked rice or cauliflower.

Tomato Dressing

Free of dairy products, wheat, yeast, corn, sugar, eggs, soy and orange.

1 cup tomato juice 1 tablespoon lemon juice 2 teaspoons finely chopped parsley 1 tablespoon finely chopped fresh basil	Combine ingredients.

Pawpaw Dressing

Free of dairy products, wheat, yeast, corn, sugar, eggs, soy, orange and nightshades.

1-2 tablespoons lemon juice 2 cups chopped ripe pawpaw	Blend ingredients. Refrigerate 1-2 hours before serving over sprouts.

Tahini Mayonnaise

Free of dairy products, wheat, corn, sugar, eggs, orange and nightshades.

4 tablespoons tahini **4 tablespoons lemon juice** **2 teaspoons honey** **2-3 teaspoons tamari or dash herbal** **seasoning** **2 teaspoons apple cider vinegar** **¼-½ teaspoon ground mustard (optional)**	Stir ingredients together well — mixture should thicken.

Olive Mayonnaise

Free of dairy products, wheat, corn, sugar, soy.
Can be made free of orange.
Can be made free of yeast by omitting tabasco.

1 egg yolk **⅓ cup cold-pressed olive oil** **1 teaspoon orange rind or lemon rind** **pinch paprika** **dash tabasco (optional)** **¼ teaspoon curry powder** **dash freshly ground black pepper** **dash herbal seasoning** **½ teaspoon onion flakes**	Beat egg yolk with a fork. Using a glass dropper add oil one drop at a time until mixture thickens. Slowly pour in remaining oil. Add other ingredients and mix well.

Olive and Lemon Dressing

Free of dairy products, wheat, yeast, corn, sugar, eggs, soy, orange and nightshades.

½ cup lemon juice **1 tablespoon olive oil** **1 teaspoon honey** **dash herbal seasoning**	Blend ingredients.

VEGETABLES

Many different combinations of vegetables and herbs can be used to create colourful and delicious dishes. Included in this section are a few ideas which we hope you will find interesting and helpful.

Baked Layered Potato Casserole

Free of dairy products, wheat, corn, sugar, eggs and orange.
Can be made free of yeast and soy by omitting tamari.

2 medium-large potatoes
2 medium onions
1 teaspoon tamari or herbal seasoning
¼ cup stock, water or soy milk
dried or fresh basil, oregano or marjoram

Slice potatoes and onions medium to thin. Layer potatoes and onions alternately in casserole dish. Add tamari to liquid and pour over casserole. Sprinkle with herbs and bake in moderate oven for ¾ hour.

Variation:

Place cooked vegetables and herbs into a dish, and top with allowable breadcrumbs.

Zucchini and Tomato

Free of dairy products, wheat, yeast, corn, sugar, eggs, soy and orange.

1 medium onion
1 cup chopped zucchini
1 cup chopped tomato
1 tablespoon chopped fresh basil
1 tablespoon chopped fresh oregano

Saute onion until transparent, add zucchini and tomato cooking until just tender. Add fresh basil and oregano.

Variation:

Place cooked vegetables and herbs into dish, top with allowable breadcrumbs and grill until browned.

Potato Chips

Free of dairy products, wheat, yeast, corn, sugar, soy, eggs and orange.

500 g potatoes	Wash potatoes well and cut into fine rounds. Dry well with tea towel or paper towel. Lightly grease oven tray and place potato pieces onto it. Bake in moderate oven 15 minutes, turn and bake a further 15 minutes. 　　Serve immediately.

Green Beans with Sesame Seeds

Free of dairy products, wheat, yeast, corn, sugar, eggs, soy, orange and nightshades.
Variation: Free of dairy products, wheat, corn, sugar, eggs, soy, orange and nightshades.

500 g green beans, sliced **¼ cup toasted sesame seeds or toasted slivered almonds**	Simmer beans until tender. Stir beans with sesame seeds. **Variation:** Serve beans cold on salads with sesame seeds and a ¼ cup apple cider vinegar mixed through.

Vegetable Spaghetti

This is a member of the squash family and is now available at most greengrocers.

1 vegetable spaghetti	Simmer spaghetti in water to cover, for 20-30 minutes. Cut in half, remove seeds and scoop out the strands of spaghetti. 　　Serve with marinara sauce or as a steamed vegetable with a protein dish.

Red Cabbage with Apple

Free of dairy products, wheat, corn, sugar, eggs, soy, orange and nightshades.
Can be made free of yeast by omitting apple cider vinegar.

½ small red cabbage, finely chopped **2 green apples, peeled and chopped** **2 tablespoons apple cider vinegar** **　　(optional)** **freshly ground black pepper**	Simmer cabbage and apples for 1 hour. Add cider vinegar and black pepper. 　　Serve with grilled fish.

Cauliflower in White Sauce
Free of dairy products, wheat, yeast, corn, sugar, eggs, soy, orange and nightshades.

1 small cauliflower, chopped into
   flowerettes
1 quantity of white sauce (see Sauces
   section)
chopped fresh parsley

Steam cauliflower until tender but not too soft. Serve with sauce. Garnish with chopped parsley and flaked almonds.

Potato Pancakes
Free of dairy products, wheat, corn, sugar, eggs and orange.
Can be made free of yeast and soy by omitting tamari.

500 g grated potato
1 small onion, finely chopped
1 tablespoon finely chopped parsley
1 tablespoon finely chopped marjoram
1 teaspoon tamari or herbal seasoning

Mix ingredients together. Drop by spoonfuls on lightly greased tray and flatten. Bake in moderate oven for 15 minutes each side or until browned.

Variation:

1 beaten egg can be added if desired.

Note: How well pancakes hold together may depend on the starchiness of the potatoes.

Spinach with Rosemary and Garlic
Free of dairy products, wheat, yeast, corn, sugar, eggs, soy, orange and nightshades.

1 small bunch spinach chopped
1-2 cloves crushed garlic
1 sprig fresh rosemary

Steam spinach with garlic and rosemary. When cooked remove rosemary and serve.

Pumpkin Balls
Free of dairy products, wheat, yeast, corn, sugar, eggs, soy, orange and nightshades.

1 medium butternut pumpkin
1 teaspoon nutmeg

Cut butternut pumpkin in half and remove seeds. Using a melon baller, scoop out balls of pumpkin. Lightly steam pumpkin balls. Place nutmeg in a tea strainer and shake over pumpkin.

   Note: Left over pumpkin can be mashed and used in soups, loaves, waffles, et cetera.

Variation:

Use potato instead of pumpkin and toss in finely chopped parsley.

Gingered Broccoli

**Free of dairy products, wheat, corn, sugar, eggs, orange and nightshades.
Can be made free of yeast and soy by omitting tamari.**

1-2 teaspoons finely chopped fresh ginger **1 bunch broccoli** **1 teaspoon honey** **1 teaspoon tamari or herbal seasoning** **¼ cup stock or water**	Saute ginger for a few minutes. Add broccoli and cook 5 minutes. Mix together honey, tamari and stock and pour over broccoli. Simmer about 5 minutes. Broccoli should not be overcooked.

Orange Carrots

Free of dairy products, wheat, yeast, corn, sugar, eggs, soy and nightshades.

2 cups sliced carrots
½ cup orange juice
2 teaspoons grated orange rind
1 tablespoon honey
2 teaspoons arrowroot or kuzu or 3
    teaspoons cornflour mixed in a
    tablespoon of water
	Cook carrots in orange juice. Add orange rind and honey. Remove carrots and keep warm. Mix arrowroot paste with orange juice and cook until thickened.
	    Serve orange sauce over carrots.

MAIN COURSES

Too often the main course of a meal is a large serving of a protein-rich food such as meat, fish or chicken with a small accompaniment of vegetables.

The most attractive and nutritious main courses are best planned along with the other parts of the meal to enable the protein-rich foods to complement and flavour the wonderful variety of vegetables and fruits available to us.

The main courses in this section offer a range of vegetarian, fish, chicken or egg dishes suitable for lunches, family dinners or entertaining.

Sweet and Sour Chicken

Free of dairy products, wheat, corn, sugar, eggs, soy, orange.　　　　*Serves 4-5*

2 onions, chopped
¼ cup chicken stock (fat skimmed off)
　or vegetable stock
1 cup chopped carrot
1 cup chopped celery
½ cup chopped capsicum
3 cups chopped cooked chicken

Sauce

2 cups pineapple juice
2 tablespoons apple cider vinegar
2 tablespoons tomato paste
2 heaped tablespoons arrowroot or kuzu
　or 3 tablespoons cornflour

Saute onions in chicken stock. Add carrot, celery and capsicum and cook 10 minutes. Add chicken. Mix ingredients for the sauce together until smooth and pour over vegetables and chicken. Simmer until sauce is thick and clear.

Serve with salad or over steamed vegetables.

Sesame Chicken

Free of dairy products, wheat, yeast, corn, sugar, eggs, soy, orange and nightshades.   *Serves 6*

4 chicken breasts or 6 fillets
½ cup allowable flour
½-¾ cup nut or soy milk
1 cup toasted sesame seeds

Remove fat and skin from chicken. Roll chicken pieces in flour. Dip in nut or soy milk. Roll in sesame seeds until coated. Bake uncovered in moderate oven until cooked.

Excellent hot or cold. Serve with sweet and sour sauce, whole baked potatoes, tabouli and coleslaw.

Chicken in Soy Sauce

Free of dairy products, wheat, sugar, eggs, orange and nightshades.
Can be made free of corn.   *Serves 4*

4 tablespoons tamari
2 tablespoons-½ cup honey
1 cup water or stock
4 tablespoons mirin or sherry
2 teaspoons fresh ginger, finely chopped
1 onion, finely chopped
1 teaspoon each cinnamon and nutmeg
1 roasting chicken, jointed with skin and
**   fat removed**
4 tablespoons arrowroot or kuzu or
**   6 tablespoons cornflour mixed with**
**   4 tablespoons water**
chopped shallots to garnish

Combine all ingredients, except chicken and arrowroot and bring to boil. Add chicken and reduce heat. Simmer approximately 45 minutes or until tender. Remove chicken and place in casserole dish. Add arrowroot, kuzu or cornflour to sauce and heat until thickened, stirring constantly. Pour sauce over chicken and garnish with chopped shallots.

Note: If cooked ahead of time and allowed to stand, the flavour will improve even more. Any fat can then be skimmed off the top of the sauce.

Serve with brown rice and lightly steamed silverbeet or snow peas and carrot straws.

Chicken and Almonds

Free of dairy products, wheat, sugar, eggs, orange and nightshades.
Can be made free of corn by omitting cornflour.   *Serves 4-6*

1 large onion
1 cup chicken stock (fat skimmed off) or
**   vegetable stock**
2 cups chopped mushrooms
2 cups chopped, cooked chicken
dash of tamari
2 teaspoons arrowroot or 3 teaspoons
**   cornflour mixed with 1 tablespoon water**
2 cups mung bean sprouts
½ cup blanched almonds, halved and
**   lightly toasted**

Saute onion in a little of the stock. Add mushrooms, chicken and tamari. Pour in remainder of stock. Make a paste with the arrowroot or cornflour and water and stir into mixture to thicken. Just before serving stir in mung beans. Garnish with almonds.

Serve with rice or noodles and tossed green salad or lightly steamed vegetables.

Note: To blanch almonds — fill a small saucepan or bowl with very hot water. Place almonds in water for a short time. Remove and slide off skins.

Chicken and Yoghurt Curry with Dhal

Free of wheat, corn, sugar, eggs, and orange.
Can be made free of dairy products and yeast by omitting yoghurt or can be made
free of soy by omitting soy milk.

Serves 4-6

Curry

1 onion, chopped

3 cloves garlic, crushed

**2 teaspoons ginger, freshly chopped or
    grated**

½ cup fresh or ¼ cup dried coriander

1 teaspoon ground turmeric

1 ½ teaspoons garam masala

chilli to taste

**½ cup non fat yoghurt or pleasant tasting
    liquid soy milk or coconut milk**

2 ripe medium tomatoes, chopped

2 cups diced, cooked chicken

Saute onion, garlic and ginger. Add coriander, turmeric and garam masala, chilli, yoghurt, coconut or soy milk and tomatoes. Cook gently for 10-15 minutes. Add chicken and simmer 5-10 minutes.

Serve with dhal, brown rice, salad and curry accompaniments.

Dhal

Free of dairy products, wheat, yeast, corn, sugar, eggs, soy, orange and nightshades.

1 large onion, finely sliced

2 cloves of garlic, crushed

2 teaspoons freshly grated ginger

½ teaspoon turmeric

1 ¼ cup red lentils (washed thoroughly)

2 ½-3 cups hot water

½ teaspoon garam masala

pinch sea salt or herbal seasoning

Saute onion, garlic and ginger. Add turmeric, stirring into mixture. Add lentils and hot water. Bring to boil, then simmer 20-30 minutes. Add garam masala and stir.

Serve with chicken curry.

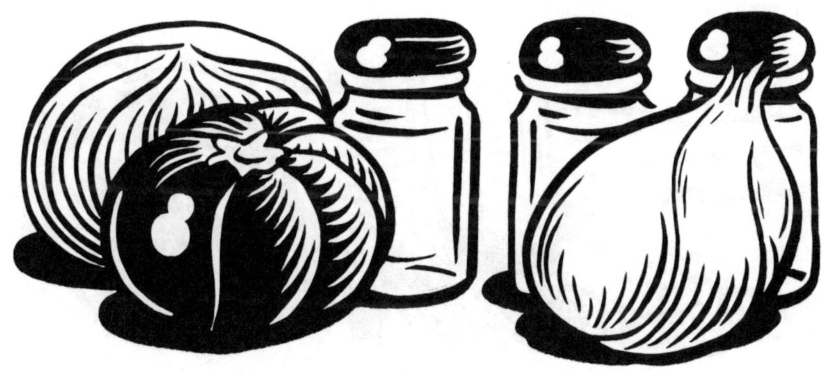

Quail or Chicken with Grapes & Macadamia Nuts

Free of dairy products, wheat, sugar, eggs, soy, orange and nightshades.
Can be made free of corn by omitting cornflour.

Serves 4

6 quail or 4-6 chicken breasts or 2 halved spatchcocks, skin removed
1 onion, chopped
2 cloves garlic, crushed
1½ cups white grape juice
½ cup vegetable stock or water
3 teaspoons apple cider vinegar
¼-½ teaspoon grated ginger
1-2 teaspoons fresh finely chopped basil
1 tablespoon chopped parsley
1 tablespoon kuzu in 2 tablespoons water or 1½ tablespoons cornflour in 3 tablespoons water
½-¾ cup roasted macadamia nuts, halved
¼-½ cup sultana grapes

Place chicken or quail in casserole. Saute onion and garlic in pan. Add juice, stock and apple cider vinegar, ginger, basil and parsley. Stir. Thicken sauce with kuzu or cornflour and pour over quail or chicken. Cook in oven approximately 45 minutes or until meat is tender. Five minutes before serving add nuts and grapes.

Serve with brown rice and green salad or choice of vegetables.

Note: To reduce fat content prepare sauce and grill or bake chicken separately. Pour over sauce and serve.

Stuffed Chicken Fillets

Free of dairy products, wheat, corn, sugar, eggs, orange and nightshade free if paprika is omitted.

Serves 4-5

10 chicken fillets, thigh or breast, all fat removed and flattened with a tenderiser
1 cup almonds, ground
2 large granny smith apples, coarsely grated
¼ cup sultanas
½-1 teaspoon tamari (or 2 teaspoons freshly chopped basil and a little apple juice to moisten nut mixture)

Combine all ingredients except chicken fillets. Spread mixture over one side of fillets. Roll fillets and lightly cover with allowable flour if desired, or sprinkle with a little paprika. Bake on greased tray approximately ½ hour in moderate oven.

Serve with pumpkin balls, broccoli and fried rice.

These can be refrigerated and thinly sliced and served as hors d'oeuvres or at luncheons.

Spatchcocks with Grapes and Macadamia Nuts (p54)

Fish Fingers (p56) and Sweet and Sour Sauce (p87)

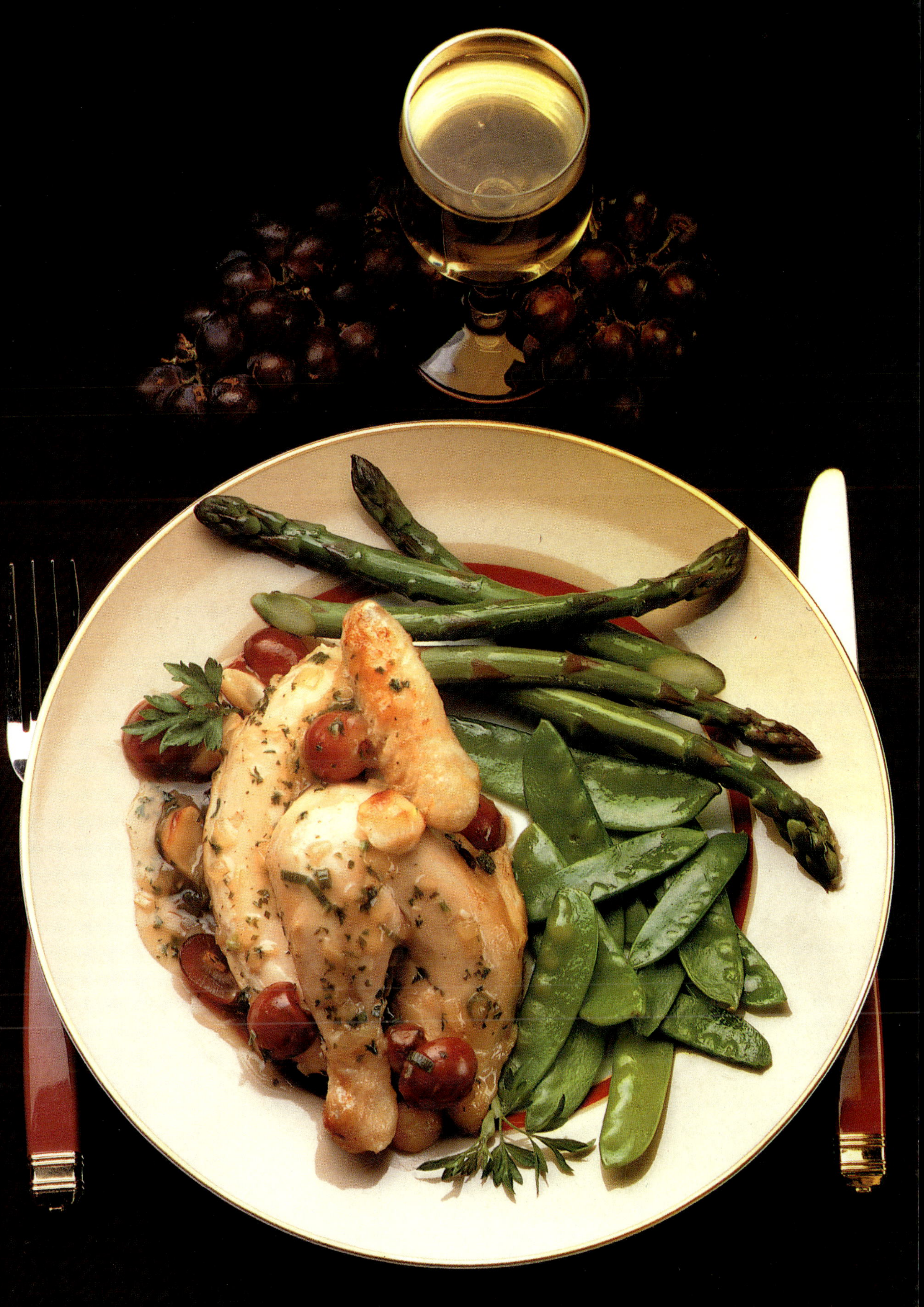

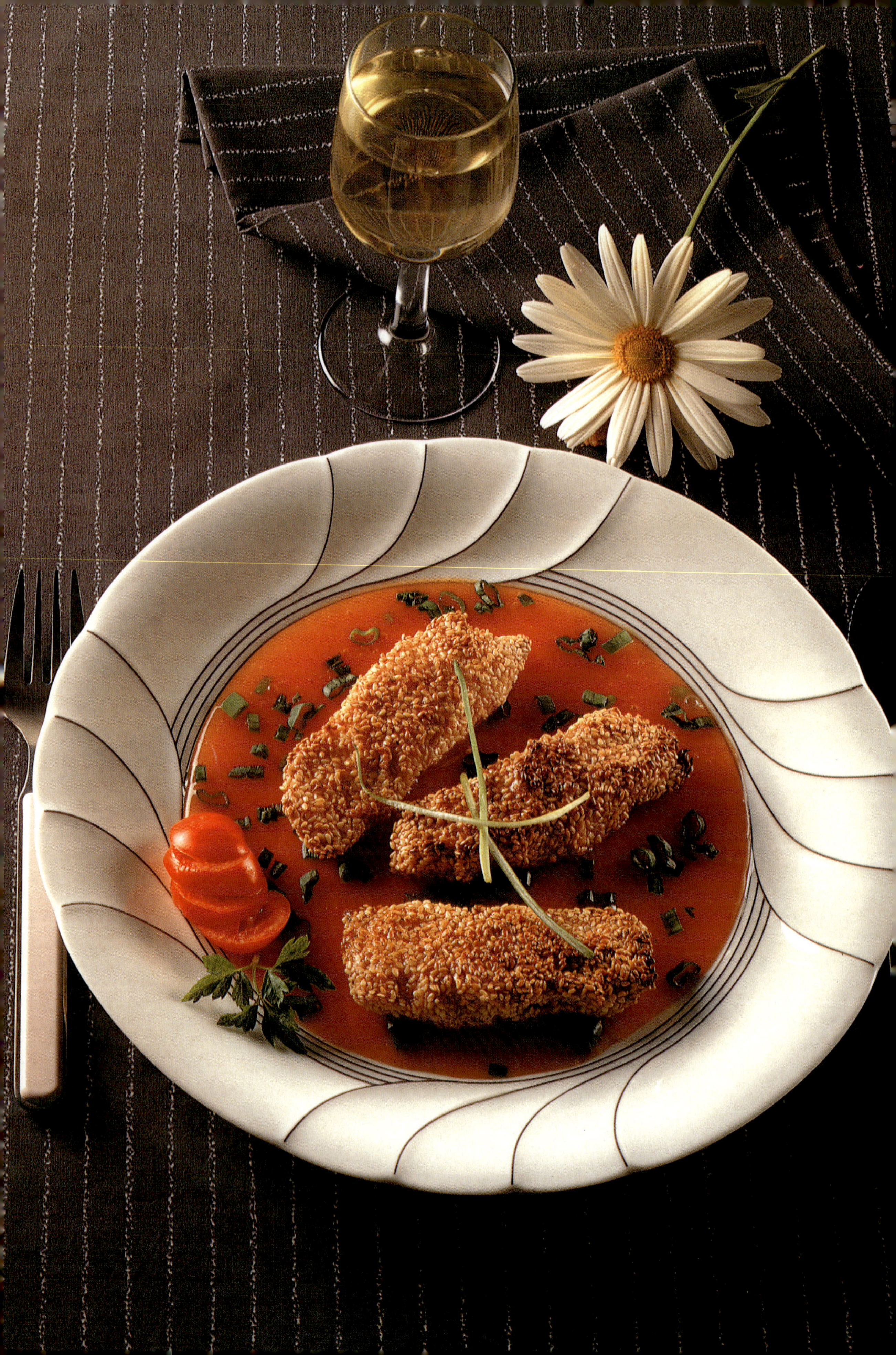

Whole Baked Schnapper

Serves 4

4 small schnapper
juice 1 lemon
lemon rings and parsley or tomato and
**   onion rings to garnish**

Stuffing (1)

Free of dairy products, wheat, corn, sugar,
eggs, soy, orange and nightshades.

1-1½ cups cooked brown rice
2 medium mushrooms, finely chopped
1 medium onion, finely chopped
1 slice of a medium-large pineapple, finely
**   chopped**
1-2 tablespoons sultanas
1/8 teaspoon five spice powder

Stuffing (2)

Free of dairy products, wheat, yeast, corn,
sugar, eggs, soy and orange.

1-1½ cups cooked brown rice
1 medium onion, finely chopped
2 tablespoons finely chopped celery
1 tablespoon finely chopped fresh basil
1 tablespoon finely chopped fresh parsley
1 finely chopped small tomato
2 teaspoons lemon rind

Combine all ingredients for stuffing of choice. Rub cavity of fish with lemon juice. Fill with stuffing. Place fish on rack in baking dish and cover with foil. Bake for ½-¾ hour in a moderate oven. Garnish with lemon rings and parsley or tomato and onion rings.

Serve with potato casserole, orange glazed carrots, spinach and cauliflower with white sauce, or your choice of salads and whole baked potato.

Sweet and Sour Casserole

Free of dairy products, wheat, corn, sugar, eggs, soy and orange.

Serves 4

2 cups chopped carrots
2 cups chopped silverbeet
1 cup chopped celery
1 medium onion, chopped
1 cup chopped zucchini
2 cloves crushed garlic
2 tablespoons fresh herbs or 1 tablespoon
**   dried e.g. basil, oregano, lovage, dill**
2 x quantity sweet and sour sauce (see
**   Sauces section)**
350 g fresh fish fillets
sufficient flour, nut milk and toasted
**   sesame seeds for coating fish**

Combine vegetables, sauce and herbs in a casserole dish. Bake in a moderate oven for 30-45 minutes. While casserole is cooking, remove skin and bones from fish, cut into bite-size pieces, then roll in flour, milk and seeds. Lightly brown fish pieces under griller. When casserole is cooked gently stir in fish pieces and serve immediately.

Serve with rice and a tossed green salad.

Fish Croquettes

Free of dairy products, wheat, yeast, corn, sugar, eggs, soy and orange.
Can be free of nightshades if sweet potato is used instead of potato and curry is omitted.   *Makes 10*

---

250 g fresh boneless fish
1-1 ½ cups mashed potato or sweet potato
1 teaspoon curry powder
1 small onion, chopped
½ tablespoon chopped parsley
½ tablespoon lemon juice
allowable breadcrumbs

Chop fish and lightly poach in a little water if desired. Flake fish and combine with remaining ingredients except breadcrumbs. Roll mixture into medium sized balls and coat with breadcrumbs. Grill until lightly browned.

Serve with grilled tomatoes, tossed salad or colourful steamed vegetables.

Fish Fingers

Free of dairy products, wheat, yeast, corn, sugar, eggs, soy, orange and nightshades.   *Serves 4*

---

500 g thick fish fillets, bones removed
½-¾ cup allowable flour
½-¾ cup nut milk or soy milk
1 ½ cups lightly toasted sesame seeds or
    finely ground almonds

Cut fish into finger shapes. Roll in flour. Dip into milk. Repeat steps two and three. Roll in sesame seeds or ground nuts till coated. Bake in a moderate oven approximately 30 minutes.

Serve with potato chips and tossed green salad.

Spaghetti Marinara

Free of dairy products, wheat, yeast, corn, sugar, eggs, soy and orange.   *Serves 4-5*

½ packet buckwheat or corn spaghetti, or
    vegetable spaghetti could be
    substituted (see Vegetables)
1 cup water
2 cups chopped tomatoes
2 tablespoons tomato paste
1 medium-large onion, chopped
2 cloves crushed garlic
2 tablespoons finely chopped parsley
½ teaspoon dried basil or 1-2 tablespoons
    fresh, chopped
3 cups fresh seafood cut into small pieces
1-2 tablespoons arrowroot or
    2 tablespoons kuzu mixed in
    2 tablespoons water

Blend water, tomatoes and tomato paste. Saute onion and garlic. Add tomato mixture to onion and garlic. Stir in parsley and basil. Stir in seafood and gently simmer until just cooked. Add arrowroot or kuzu paste, stirring till thickened. Pour over cooked spaghetti and serve immediately.

Serve with green salad.

Fish Fillets with Curry Sauce and Mango

Free of dairy products, wheat, corn, sugar, eggs, soy and orange.
Can be free of yeast if sultanas are omitted.
Can be made free of corn if cornflour is omitted.

Serves 4

1 onion, finely chopped
½ teaspoon garam masala
½ teaspoon ground coriander
½-1 teaspoon curry powder (or to taste)
1-2 tablespoons tomato paste
1 cup coconut milk
2 tablespoons sultanas (optional)
1 tablespoon kuzu mixed in 1 tablespoon
     water or 1 ½ tablespoons cornflour
     mixed in 2 tablespoons water
1 large mango chopped into bite size
     pieces
4 fish fillets, e.g. ocean perch, gemfish or
     bream, sprinkled with 2 tablespoons
     lemon juice

Saute onion. Add garam masala, coriander and curry powder. Saute about a minute, stirring well. Stir in tomato paste. Add coconut milk and stir well. Add sultanas and simmer. Add kuzu or cornflour paste, stirring till thickened. Add mango. Lightly grill fish fillets. Spoon sauce over fillets and serve immediately.

Serve with the following accompaniments: cucumber in yoghurt or cucumber sprinkled with basil or dill, chopped banana rolled in coconut or tomato and onion rings and green salad.

Cabbage Rolls

Free of dairy products, wheat, corn, sugar, eggs, orange.
Can be made free of yeast and soy if tamari is omitted.

Makes 10

1 ½ cups cooked brown rice
2 cloves crushed garlic
1 tomato, finely chopped
1 stick finely chopped celery
1 tablespoon chopped fresh basil
1 tablespoon chopped fresh oregano
3 shallots, chopped
2 medium boneless fish fillets, cut into
     very small pieces
dash tamari (optional) or herbal seasoning
¼ cup fresh tomato juice
1 tablespoon tomato paste
Chinese cabbage leaves, washed
cotton or string for tying rolls

Combine all ingredients, except cabbage leaves. Place spoonfuls of mixture onto leaves and roll into a parcel. Tie with cotton or string to hold together. Steam or bake until cooked. Remove cotton or string.

Serve with yellow and green vegetables.

Savoury Lentils

Free of dairy products, wheat, yeast, corn, sugar, eggs and orange.   *Serves 3-4*

1 cup brown lentils, washed thoroughly
2 cups water
1 medium onion, chopped
1 cup chopped carrot
1 cup chopped swede or parsnip
½ cup peas
1 tablespoon tomato paste
dash tamari (optional)

Place all ingredients in a saucepan. Bring to the boil, then simmer 30-40 minutes.

Serve with brown rice, spinach and carrots.

Lentil Shepherd's Pie

Free of dairy products, wheat, yeast, corn, sugar, eggs, soy and orange.   *Serves 4-5*

1 quantity cooked savoury lentils (see
    above recipe)
1 kg potatoes, peeled, or substitute sweet
    potato or pumpkin
pinch sea salt (optional)

Place lentils in a casserole dish. Cook potatoes till soft. Drain potatoes, then mash with a little hot water or vegetable stock. Add sea salt if desired, then spread over lentils. Bake in oven till hot.

Serve with green beans, pumpkin, zucchini and tomatoes.

Hiziki with Vegetables and Tofu

Free of dairy product, wheat, corn, sugar, eggs, orange and nightshades.   *Serves 4-5*

40 g hiziki sea vegetable, soaked in water
    to cover for ½ hour
3 cups diced vegetables, e.g. carrot, onion,
    celery
2 cups diced tofu
¼ cup water or stock
1 tablespoon honey
1 tablespoon tamari

Drain hiziki and rinse well. Saute vegetables for 5 minutes. Add hiziki, tofu, water or stock, honey and tamari and simmer for 10 minutes.

Serve with brown rice and mixed salad or orange sweet potato and mixed salad.

Millet Casserole

Free of dairy products, wheat, corn, sugar, eggs and orange.
Can be made free of soy if tamari is omitted.

Serves 4-6

2 onions, sliced

2 cloves crushed garlic

1 cup hulled millet

3 ½ cups vegetable stock

1 cup carrot juice

2 bay leaves

1 tablespoon tomato paste

½-1 tablespoon tamari (optional) or herbal
seasoning

2 cups sliced mushrooms

2 cups sliced carrots

Place all ingredients in a deep round casserole dish with a tight-fitting lid. Bake in a moderate oven for approximately 2 hours or until all the liquid is absorbed. Remove bay leaves before serving.

Serve with a variety of green vegetables.

Corn Fritters

Free of dairy products, wheat, sugar, eggs, orange and nightshades.
Can be made free of yeast and soy if tamari is omitted.

Makes 12

¾ cup brown rice flour

¼ teaspoon bicarb soda

1 cup ground almonds

1 teaspoon mixed herbs

¾ cup soy or nut milk mixed with

3 teaspoons kuzu, arrowroot or
½ cup soy or nut milk mixed with
1 beaten egg

3 shallots, chopped

3 cobs cooked corn, then corn cut off the
cobs

dash tamari or herbal seasoning

Mix all ingredients together. Place spoonfuls under griller and brown lightly, then turn.

Serve with mushroom sauce, waldorf salad, sprout salad and carrot and raisin salad.

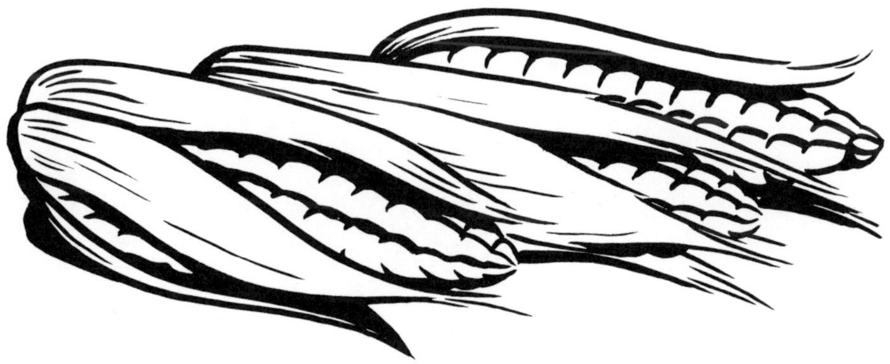

Baked Beans

Free of dairy products, wheat, corn, sugar, eggs and orange.
Can be made free of yeast and soy if tamari is omitted.

Serves 4-6

1¾ cups haricot beans, soaked overnight
1 medium onion, chopped
2 cloves crushed garlic
2 medium tomatoes, chopped
2½-3 cups vegetable stock or water
1-2 teaspoons honey
2 teaspoons molasses
½ teaspoon curry powder
½-1 teaspoon ground mustard
1 tablespoon tamari (optional) or herbal
   seasoning
2 tablespoons tomato paste
a little potato flour to thicken if necessary

Drain beans and place in a casserole dish. Add remaining ingredients. Bake in a low-moderate oven for approximately 3-4 hours or until beans are soft and have absorbed the colour. When cooked, check the consistency of the beans. If the mixture is too thick, add a little more water. If too liquid, sprinkle with potato flour to thicken.

Serve with toasted or baked seed bread (see Bread section) or chappatis and salad for a tasty lunch.

Chick Pea Loaf

Free of dairy products, wheat, yeast, corn, sugar, soy and orange.
Can be free of nightshades if tomato juice omitted.

Serves 4-6

1 cup chick peas
2 cups vegetable stock or tomato juice or a
   mixture
¾ cup ground walnuts
1 cup rolled millet
1 cup finely chopped onion
1 cup finely chopped celery
½ cup finely chopped parsley
1 beaten egg or 2 egg whites
2 tablespoons sesame seeds

Soak chick peas overnight. Drain and rinse well, then cover with fresh water and cook 1 hour or until tender. Drain and mash or place in blender with stock and/or juice. Blend and pour into basin. Mix in remaining ingredients and pour into a lightly greased loaf tin. Sprinkle sesame seeds on top and bake in a moderate oven about 45 minutes. Allow to cool a little before turning out of tin, then slice thickly and serve with tomato sauce.

Serve with green beans and pumpkin balls.

Nut Terrine

Free of dairy products, wheat, corn, sugar, eggs, orange and nightshades.   *Serves 8-10*

1½ **cups chopped onion**
1½ **cups chopped celery**
2-3 cloves crushed garlic
½ **cup chopped walnuts**
1 cup almonds, ground
1 cup chopped toasted cashews
¼ **cup rolled millet**
1 tablespoon chopped parsley or chives
½ **teaspoon dried or 1 tablespoon chopped**
     fresh basil
200 g tofu, mashed
¾ **cup mashed steamed pumpkin**
1 tablespoon tamari (optional)
1 tablespoon sesame seeds, to garnish

Saute onion, celery and garlic. Add nuts, millet and herbs. Blend tofu, pumpkin and tamari and combine with other ingredients. Spoon into a lightly greased loaf tin. Sprinkle with sesame seeds and bake in a moderate oven for 45 minutes or until firm. Remove from oven and cool slightly before turning out.

This terrine makes an excellent luncheon dish with an assortment of salads.

Carrot and Nut Loaf

Free of dairy products, wheat, yeast, corn, sugar, soy and orange.   *Serves 4*

2 cups grated carrot
1½ **cups cooked brown rice**
1½ **cups ground walnuts or cashews**
1 finely chopped onion
¼ **cup finely chopped capsicum**
¼ **cup finely chopped celery**
2 tablespoons finely chopped parsley
2 teaspoons lemon juice
1 large beaten egg or 2 stiffly beaten egg
     whites

Mix all ingredients together. Pour into a lightly greased loaf tin and bake in a moderate oven until firm. Leave to cool a little, then cut into thick slices.

Serve with tossed green salad, sprouts and beetroot salad or lightly steamed vegetables.

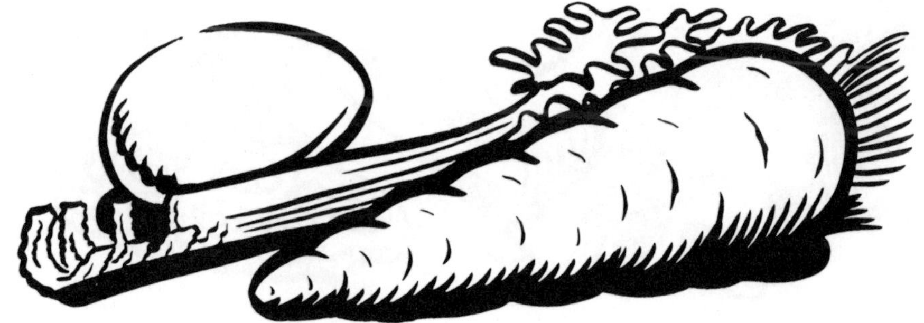

Vegetarian Rolls

Free of dairy products, wheat, corn, sugar, eggs and orange.
Can be made free of yeast if tamari is omitted.

Makes 16

Pastry

1 cup soy flour
1 cup buckwheat flour
½ cup potato flour
1 cup water

Filling

3 cups dry mashed potato
1 ½ cups ground almonds
3 tablespoons finely chopped capsicum
1 tablespoon chopped chives or shallots
1 tablespoon finely chopped fresh basil
1 ½ teaspoons cummin
1-1 ½ teaspoons curry powder
dash tamari or herbal seasoning
3 tablespoons finely chopped parsley

Mix dry ingredients together. Add water and mix into a firm ball. Knead lightly and refrigerate for 30 minutes or while preparing filling.

Mix together ingredients for filling. Cut pastry into four equal parts. On a well-floured bench or board (potato flour is useful for this), roll out 1 part pastry into a rectangle 28 x 11-12 cm with a long edge running from left to right. Place 1 cup well packed filling onto pastry, roll into a log shape as long as the pastry, then place on nearer long edge of pastry. Roll pastry over to wrap up filling. Cut into 4 x 7 cm lengths. Repeat with remaining 3 parts pastry and filling. Place rolls onto a lightly greased tray and bake in a moderately slow oven till crisp and lightly browned.

Serve with tomato sauce, green salad, coleslaw and sprouts.

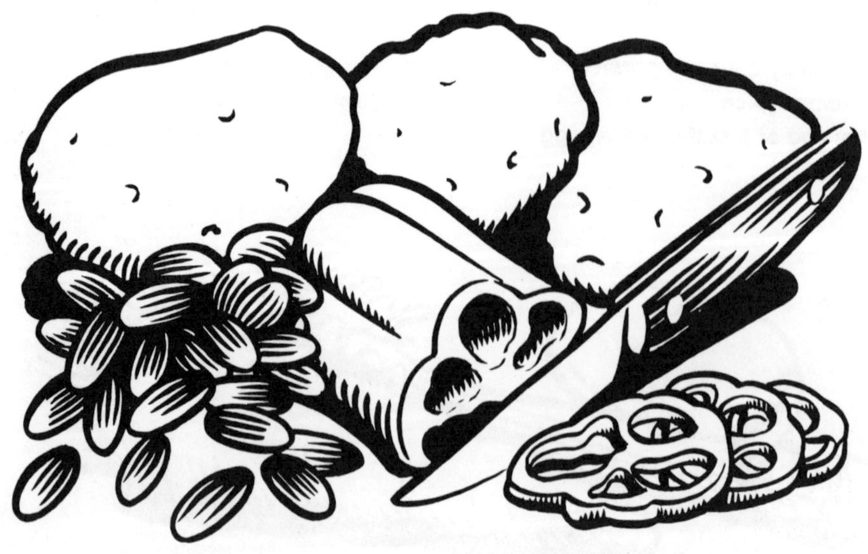

Vegetable Pasties

Free of wheat, corn, sugar, eggs and orange.
Can be made free of dairy if cottage cheese is omitted.
Can be made free of yeast if tamari, mushrooms and tofu are omitted.   *Makes 8*

Pastry

**1 quantity sausage roll pastry (see above
    recipe)**

Filling

**2 cups steamed vegetables, e.g. potato,
    pumpkin, green beans, peas, carrot,
    parsnip**
1 clove crushed garlic
1 medium-large onion, finely chopped
**1 cup chopped mushrooms or use an extra
    cup steamed vegetables**
**½ cup cooked lentils or crumbled tofu or
    cottage cheese**
2 tablespoons tomato paste
2 tablespoons finely chopped fresh basil
**1 tablespoon tamari (optional) or herbal
    seasoning**

Roll out pastry on a well-floured board or bench. Cut out in circles approximately 14-15 cm in diameter — a saucer is useful for this.

Combine vegetables, garlic, onion and mushrooms and mash well. Add lentils, tofu or cottage cheese, tomato paste, basil and tamari. Place a heaped tablespoonful of the mixture onto each pastry circle, being careful to fill the pastry from end to end while leaving room for joining ends. Pinch each circle together at the top or on the side by folding the pastry over. Prick with a fork on the sides. Bake on a greased tray until crisp and lightly browned.

Serve with green salad, sprouts and carrot and raisin salad.

Buckwheat Rissoles

Free of dairy products, wheat, sugar, eggs, corn, orange and nightshades.
Can be made free of yeast and soy if tamari is omitted.   *Serves 4-6*

1 cup buckwheat groats
1½ cups water
1 small onion, finely chopped
¼ cup very finely chopped carrot
¼ cup very finely chopped celery
**1-2 teaspoons finely chopped or grated
    fresh ginger**
1 clove crushed garlic
dash tamari or herbal seasoning
1 tablespoon finely chopped shallots
1-2 teaspoons finely chopped fresh basil
**2-3 teaspoons kuzu, cornflour or arrowroot
    mixed in 1 tablespoon water**
**sufficient sesame seeds for coating
    rissoles**

Cook buckwheat in water until all the liquid has been absorbed. Add remaining ingredients immediately while buckwheat is still warm, except sesame seeds. Shape into small rissoles and roll in sesame seeds. Cook in a small amount of ghee or place under the griller.

Serve with purple salad, green salad and carrot and raisin salad. Mushroom or tomato sauce (see Sauces) complement these rissoles.

Hazelnut and Potato Rissoles

Free of dairy products, wheat, corn, sugar, eggs, soy and oranges.   *Serves 4-6*

2 medium onions, chopped
2 cloves garlic, crushed
½ cup chopped mushrooms
2 cups mashed steamed potato (with skin
   on)
2 cups ground hazelnuts
1 tablespoon chopped fresh basil

Saute onion and garlic. Add mushrooms and cook briefly. Combine all ingredients in a bowl. Shape into patties and roll in coarse polenta or allowable flour. Bake on a lightly greased tray or heat under griller.

Serve with coleslaw, waldorf salad and beetroot salad.

Quiche

Free of dairy products, wheat, sugar and orange.
Can be made free of yeast if mushrooms and tamari are omitted.
Can be made free of soy if tamari and soy milk are omitted.   *Serves 4-6*

Base

¾ cup barley flour
¾ cup ground pecans
⅓-½ cup water

Filling

3 eggs
1 cup pleasant tasting liquid soy milk or
   thick nut milk
1 cup chopped mushrooms or 1 cup corn
   kernels
1 cup chopped spinach
1 cup chopped steamed asparagus
½ cup chopped onion
¼ teaspoon nutmeg
1-2 drops tabasco sauce
1 tablespoon tamari or sprinkle herbal
   seasoning (optional)
1 tablespoon tomato paste
1 tablespoon lemon juice
1 tablespoon brown rice flour
dash freshly ground black pepper

Mix all ingredients together in a bowl. Lightly grease a pie dish and press base onto this. Bake in moderate oven 10 minutes, do not brown. Allow to cool before adding filling.

Beat eggs with milk. Add remaining ingredients. Pour over base and bake in a moderate oven for 30-40 minutes.

Serve with a tossed green salad.

Hiziki Pie

Free of dairy products, wheat, corn, sugar, eggs, orange and nightshades.
Can be free of yeast and soy if tamari is omitted.

Serves 4

Base

¾ cup brown rice flour
¾ cup rolled millet
5-6 tablespoons water

Mix all ingredients together. Press onto lightly greased pie plate.

Filling

⅓-½ cup dried hiziki, soaked for ½ hour,
    drained and then rinsed
2 onions, chopped
2 cloves garlic, crushed
1 teaspoon chopped fresh ginger
2 cups diced pumpkin
2 cups mixed chopped vegetables
dash tamari or herbal seasoning (optional)
2 teaspoons chopped fresh basil

Saute onions, garlic and ginger. Add pumpkin and other vegetables and simmer until soft. Drain off vegetable liquid (use for soups etc). Mash vegetables, adding tamari, basil and hiziki. Spoon onto crust and bake in moderate oven 20-30 minutes.

Serve with garden fresh peas and mint, carrot straws and broccoli.

Spinach Pie

Free of dairy products, wheat, yeast, corn, sugar, soy, orange and nightshades.

Serves 3-4

Base

¾ cup rolled millet
¾ cup brown rice flour
5-6 tablespoons water

Combine all ingredients and press onto a lightly greased pie plate.

Filling

1 large onion, finely chopped
1 cup cooked mashed pumpkin
2 cups lightly steamed spinach
pinch nutmeg
½-¾ cup ground almonds or other nuts
3 beaten eggs

Saute onion, then place in bowl. Add pumpkin, spinach, nutmeg and nuts. Lastly add eggs and mix well. Pour over base and cook in a moderate oven for 45 minutes.

Serve with tabouli salad and hot roasted potatoes.

Savoury Lima Beans

Free of dairy products, wheat, corn, sugar, eggs and orange.
Can be made free of yeast and soy if tamari is omitted.

Serves 4

1½ cups lima beans
1 large onion, chopped
2-3 cloves crushed garlic
1 tablespoon tomato paste
2 medium-large cooking tomatoes,
   chopped
dash tamari or herbal seasoning
freshly chopped basil and parsley

Soak beans overnight, then drain. Plunge beans into boiling water, then simmer until soft. Saute onion and garlic. Stir in tomato paste, tomatoes, tamari and drained beans. Simmer 10-15 minutes, then stir in basil and parsley.

Should you forget to soak the beans, an alternative method is:

Bring water to boil, add the beans and boil one minute. Remove from heat, allow to stand for 30 minutes. Boil and simmer till tender. Now continue from sauteing onions.

Other vegetables such as chopped celery, carrot, parsnip and capsicum can be added. If mixture is too thick add a little water or stock.

Serve with broccoli, carrots and potato casserole.

Vegetable Crumble

Free of dairy products, wheat, corn, sugar, eggs and orange.
Can be made free of yeast and soy if tamari is omitted.

Serves 6

Topping

½ cup ground pecans
½ cup buckwheat flour
½ cup millet flour
1 tablespoon chives
¼ cup chopped shallots
1 tablespoon fresh basil
½ teaspoon mixed herbs
1 tablespoon tamari or herbal seasoning
⅓ cup water

Mix all ingredients together except water. Add water and mix well.

Filling

1 cup brown lentils cooked with
   1 teaspoon of tumeric
6 cups chopped mixed vegetables
¾ cup water mixed with 1 tablespoon
   tomato paste

Mix all ingredients together. Pour into base of casserole dish or large pie dish. Crumble topping over filling. Bake in moderate oven 30-45 minutes or until topping is brown.

Tofu Casserole

Free of dairy products, wheat, corn, sugar, eggs and orange.   *Serves 4*

1 medium onion, chopped
2 cloves garlic, crushed
400 g tofu, cut into 2cm cubes
¼ cup allowable flour in plastic bag
1 teaspoon mixed herbs
¼-½ cup tomato paste
1 cup water
2 medium tomatoes, chopped
1 teaspoon basil, chopped
1 teaspoon chives, chopped
1 cup chopped cauliflower
½ cup peas

Lightly saute onion and garlic and place in casserole dish. Place tofu in bag with flour and shake to coat, then add to casserole. Add all other ingredients and mix well together. Bake in moderate oven for 30-45 minutes. Serve with noodles or rice and steamed broccoli.

Tofu Curry

Free of dairy products, wheat, corn, sugar, eggs, orange and nightshades.   *Serves 4*

1 medium large onion, chopped
1-2 cloves garlic, crushed
½-1 teaspoon grated fresh ginger
1 teaspoon-1 tablespoon or more of curry
powder to taste
½ teaspoon cummin
½ teaspoon coriander
½ teaspoon garam masala
2 cups liquid — 1 cup coconut milk and
1 cup vegetable stock (or ½ cup
vegetable stock and ½ cup fruit or
vegetable juice)
2 tablespoons red lentils
stick cinnamon
½ cup sultanas or cooked garbanzos
400 g tofu, cubed

Saute onion, garlic and all spices except cinnamon. Add liquid, then lentils, cinnamon and sultanas or garbanzos. Simmer gently until lentils are very soft and thickening the liquid. Add tofu and heat through.

Serve with brown rice, cucumber in yoghurt and carraway seeds, chappatis or pappadams and green salad.

Note: This curry will improve in flavour if allowed to stand before eating.

Pizza

Free of dairy products, wheat, corn, sugar, eggs and orange.   *Serves 4*

Base

¾ cup buckwheat flour
¾ cup brown rice flour
½ teaspoon bicarbonate of soda
1 teaspoon cream of tartar
½ cup water

Mix dry ingredients together. Add water and mix thoroughly. Press with fork onto lightly greased pizza plate.

Topping

3 tablespoons tomato paste
300 g mashed tofu
1 large onion, chopped
2 cloves garlic, crushed
3 medium tomatoes, sliced
2 tablespoons chopped fresh basil or
   ¼ tablespoon dried
1 tablespoon chopped fresh oregano or
   ¼ teaspoon dried
1 cup sliced medium mushrooms
¾ cup chopped green capsicum

Mash tofu with tomato paste and spread over the base. Saute onions and garlic and spread over tofu and tomato. Add sliced tomato. Sprinkle with herbs, mushrooms and capsicum. Bake in a moderate oven for 30 minutes or longer.

Serve with tossed green salad.

Raw Nut Mould

Free of dairy products, wheat, yeast, corn, sugar, eggs, soy, orange and nightshades.   *Serves 4*

1 cup ground almonds
1-1 ½ cups ground cashews
½-1 large carrot grated
1 stick celery, chopped
juice 1 lemon
juice 1 orange or ¼ cup carrot juice

Mix all ingredients, adding juice last. Use sufficient only to enable mixture to hold together. Place in small basin to mould shape. Invert basin and serve on lettuce leaves with tomato wedges. Garnish with thin slices of mushrooms, tomatoes and parsley sprigs.

Serve with purple salad, buckwheat lettuce, tomato, onion and cucumber.

Raw Patties

Free of dairy products, wheat, yeast, corn, sugar, eggs, soy, orange and nightshades.　　　*Serves 4*

1 avocado
1 cup almonds or pecans, ground
1 onion, finely chopped
1 stick celery, finely chopped
1 tablespoon fresh sage or basil
1 tablespoon chopped parsley
1 tablespoon chopped chives
squeeze lemon juice

Mash avocado and mix with remaining ingredients. Form into patties using two spoons. Serve on lettuce leaves garnished with chopped red capsicum.

Vegetarian Fried Rice

Free of dairy products, wheat, yeast, sugar, eggs, soy and orange.　　　*Serves 4-6*

1 large onion, chopped
2 cloves garlic, crushed
½ cup finely diced carrot
½ cup finely chopped celery
¼ cup finely chopped red capsicum
½ cup cooked peas
½ cup corn kernels
1 apple, peeled and chopped
3 cups cooked brown rice
2 tablespoons finely chopped parsley
1 teaspoon curry powder or cummin (optional)
toasted sesame seeds or chopped roasted nuts

Saute onion, garlic, carrot and celery for 5 minutes. Add capsicum, peas, corn and apple, cook a further 5 minutes. Stir in rice, parsley and curry powder and continue cooking until rice is hot. Garnish with seeds or nuts and chopped shallots.

Serve with grilled mushrooms and lightly steamed vegetables or green salad.

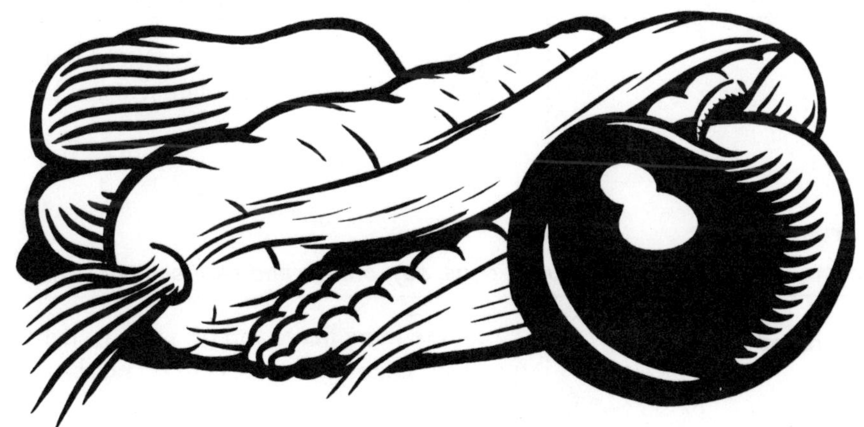

DESSERTS AND CREAMS

The ideal dessert is fresh fruit in season. However, as most people enjoy a wide range of desserts, we have provided a variety of wholesome and delicious ones. Many of these are our family favourites.

Pie Crusts

Nut Crust

Free of dairy products, wheat, yeast, corn, sugar, eggs, soy, orange and nightshades.

1½ cups ground almonds **½ cup ground pecans**	Combine nuts and press over pie plate ready to fill.

Coconut/Nut Crust

Free of dairy products, wheat, yeast, corn, sugar, eggs, soy, orange and nightshades.

½ cup coconut **½ cup pecans, ground** **1 cup almonds, ground**	Combine ingredients and press over pie plate. Bake blind in a moderate oven for 10 minutes, or leave unbaked, depending on recipe.

Millet/Coconut Crust

Free of dairy products, wheat, yeast, corn, sugar, eggs, soy, orange and nightshades.

½ cup brown rice flour **½ cup rolled millet** **½ cup coconut** **4 tablespoons water**	Combine grains and coconut. Mix in water and press onto a lightly greased pie plate. Do not bake before filling.

Pecan/Barley Crust

Free of dairy products, wheat, yeast, corn, sugar, eggs, soy, orange and nightshades.

¾ cup pecan nuts, ground **¾ cup barley flour** **⅓ cup water**	Combine ingredients and press into a lightly greased pie dish. Bake 10 minutes but do not brown.

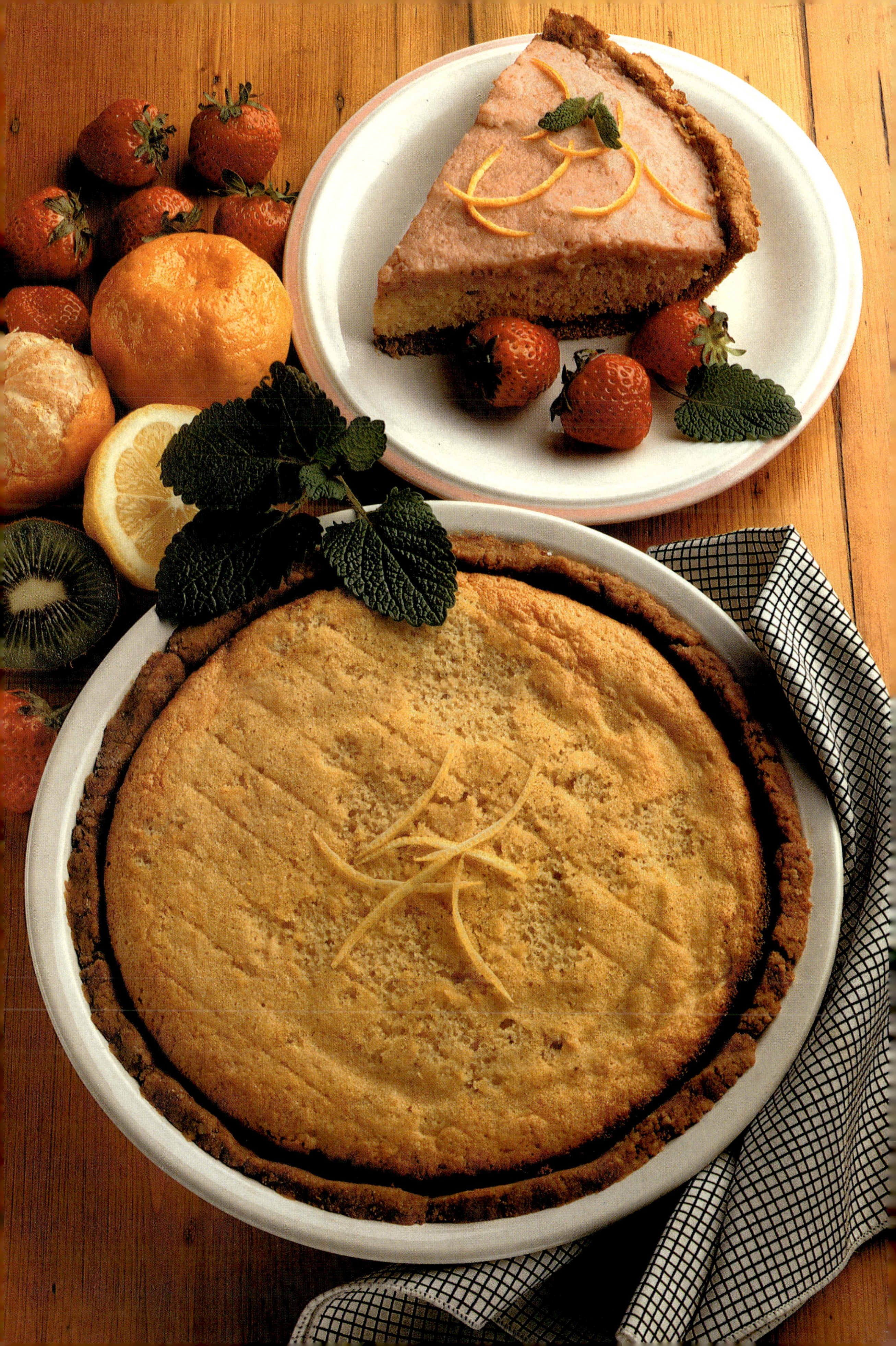

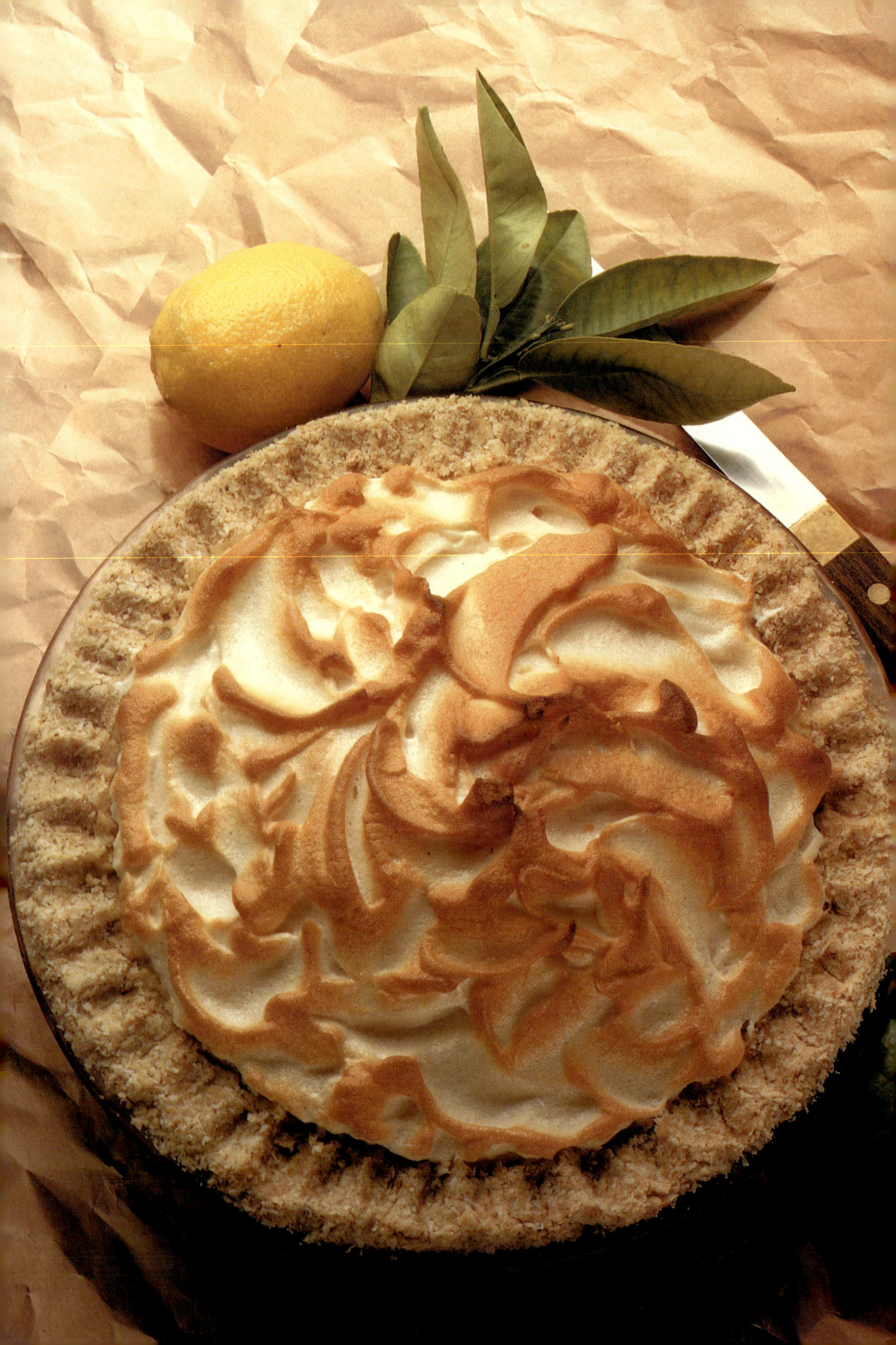

Nutty Rice Crust

Free of dairy products, wheat, yeast, corn, sugar, eggs, soy, orange and nightshades.

½ **cup brown rice flour** ½ **cup pecans, ground** ½ **cup coconut** ⅓ **cup water**	Combine and press into a lightly greased tray. Bake 15 minutes so that lightly browned or leave unbaked, depending on recipe.

Lemon Meringue Pie

Free of dairy products, wheat, yeast, corn, sugar, soy, orange and nightshades. *Serves 6*

Base

Nutty rice crust, baked.

Cool before adding filling.

Filling

2 tablespoons agar* flakes
½ **cup apple juice**
½ **cup water**
¼-½ **cup honey**
2 tablespoons arrowroot or 3 tablespoons cornflour
½ **cup lemon juice**
2 teaspoons lemon rind
1 cup soy milk or thick nut milk

Soak agar in apple juice, water and honey. Bring to the boil and simmer till flakes have dissolved. Mix arrowroot or cornflour with lemon juice and add to agar mixture, stiring over a low heat until mixture has thickened slightly. Remove from heat and add rind and milk, mixing well. When the mixture has cooled and is beginning to set spoon gently over the crust and leave until completely set before adding the topping. Placing in the refrigerator or freezer will speed up this process.

Topping

2 egg whites
pinch cream of tartar
2 tablespoons maple syrup

Beat egg whites with cream of tartar till stiff. Slowly add maple syrup and continue beating. Spread over pie, forming peaks, and bake in a hot oven for 5 minutes. Turn the oven off, open the door and allow to cool.

* See note on agar in Glossary.

Strawberry Sponge Shortcake (p83)

Lemon Meringue Pie (p71)

Pumpkin Pie

Free of dairy products, wheat, corn, sugar, eggs, orange and nightshades. *Serves 6-8*

Base

Nut crust or coconut/nut crust, unbaked

Filling

2 cups cold dry mashed steamed pumpkin
½ cup honey
2 cups mashed tofu
4 tablespoons lemon juice
rind 1 lemon
½-1 teaspoon ground ginger
2 teaspoons ground cinnamon

Blend all ingredients. Spread over base and bake in moderate oven 30-40 minutes. Cool and chill. The longer this pie is refrigerated, the more the flavour and texture will improve.

Serve with cashew cream or tofu cream.

No-bake Strawberry Slice or Cheesecake

Free of dairy products, wheat, corn, sugar, eggs, orange and nightshades. *Serves 5-6*

Base

Nut crust or coconut/nut crust, baked

Filling

1 cup apple juice
2 tablespoons agar* flakes
2 cups mashed tofu
1½ cups pureed strawberries
1-2 tablespoons honey

Soak agar flakes in apple juice overnight or for 1-2 hours. Blend tofu, strawberries and honey. Bring agar mixture to the boil and simmer until flakes have dissolved. Stir into tofu mixture and pour over base. Decorate with fresh strawberries and place in refrigerator to set.

* See note on agar in Glossary.

Lemon Cheesecake

Free of dairy products, wheat, corn, sugar, orange and nightshades. *Serves 6*

Crust

Nut crust, or coconut/nut crust, unbaked

Filling

3 cups mashed tofu
rind of 1 lemon
⅓ cup lemon juice
½ cup honey
2 eggs, separated

Blend tofu, lemon rind and juice, honey and egg yolks. Beat egg whites till stiff and gently fold into mixture. Spoon over crust and bake in a moderate oven until set. Cool, then refrigerate.

Serve garnished with fresh strawberries or kiwi fruit.

Ginger, Pumpkin and Date Pie

Free of dairy products, wheat, yeast, corn, sugar, soy, orange and nightshades.   *Serves 5-6*

Base

Pecan/barley crust

Filling

2 eggs
¾ cup soy or nut milk
1 teaspoon ground ginger
½ teaspoon cinnamon
¼ teaspoon mixed spice
1 tablespoon-¼ cup honey
1 ½ cups mashed cooked pumpkin
1 tablespoon barley flour to thicken
¼ cup chopped fresh dates

Blend all ingredients and pour into pie shell. Bake in a moderate oven 35-40 minutes or until set.
   Serve with nut cream or tofu cream.

Apple Pie

Free of dairy products, wheat, yeast, corn, sugar, eggs, soy, orange and nightshades.   *Serves 4-6*

Base

Nut crust or coconut/nut crust, baked

Filling

4 large or 6 medium Granny Smith apples,
    peeled and chopped
6 cloves or ¼ teaspoon, ground
1 tablespoon-¼ cup honey
stick cinnamon
a little water to cover bottom of saucepan
strip lemon rind
1 teaspoon ground cinnamon

Place all ingredients except ground cinnamon in saucepan. Heat and gently simmer until apples are soft and remove cinnamon stick. Pour into pie crust and dust with cinnamon. Bake in a moderate oven for 20-30 minutes.

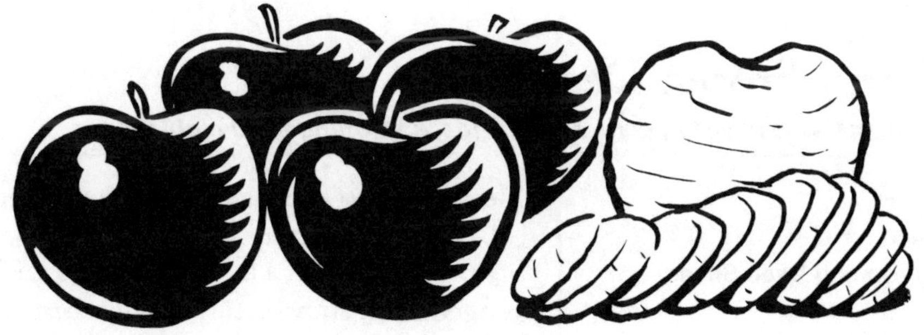

Ricotta Cheesecake

Free of wheat, corn, sugar, soy, orange and nightshades. *Serves 6-8*

Base

**Nutty-rice crust, unbaked and pressed into
a lightly greased springform pan.**

Filling

**3 cups firm ricotta cheese, or a mixture of
ricotta cheese and cottage cheese**
4 eggs
¾ cup yoghurt
½ cup honey
⅓ cup lemon juice
rind 1 lemon
few drops pure vanilla
pulp 3 passionfruit

Blend all ingredients except passionfruit. Pour into crust and bake in a moderate oven until set. Cool, then refrigerate. Spread passionfruit over cheesecake. Serve with fresh fruit salad.

Orange Sherbet

Free of dairy products, wheat, yeast, corn, sugar, eggs, soy and nightshades. *Serves 8*

8 juicy oranges
2 tablespoons agar* flakes
2 cups almond milk
2-4 tablespoons maple syrup
½-1 tablespoon orange rind

Cut the top quarter off each of 8 oranges. Carefully scoop out the orange pulp from the oranges without damaging the skins. Place orange shells in fridge. Squeeze the juice from the pulp to make 2 cups. Soak agar flakes in orange juice for 1-2 hours. Heat agar/orange mixture gently until flakes have dissolved. Blend agar/orange mixture with remaining ingredients. Pour into a tray and freeze until hard around the edges. Blend again, repour into tray and freeze. When frozen, cut into squares and place in orange shells.

    *See note on agar in Glossary.

Banana-berry Frozen Dessert

Free of dairy products, wheat, yeast, corn, sugar, eggs, soy, orange and nightshades. *Serves 4-5*

6 medium bananas
¼ cup lemon juice
**1 quantity berry topping *(see Slices
section)**

Blend bananas and lemon juice and freeze in a 20 cm cake tin. The mixture should be approximately 2½ cm high. When frozen add berry topping and refreeze.

    Serve with strawberries or other berries.

    * Any leftover topping can be used on waffles.

Strawberry Icecream

Free of dairy products, wheat, yeast, corn, sugar, eggs, soy, orange and nightshades.　　*Serves 4-5*

2 punnets strawberries (500 g)
2 medium bananas
1 avocado
¼ cup honey
½ cup orange juice or 2 tablespoons tahini
**   (the tahini will give a creamier texture**
**   than the orange juice)**

Blend all ingredients at high speed. Pour into a container and freeze.

Variation:

Use only 1 cup strawberries and replace the other punnet with 1 cup fresh or frozen raspberries.
    Serve with fresh fruit salad.

Carob Icecream

Free of dairy products, wheat, corn, sugar, eggs, soy, orange and nightshades.　　*Serves 4-6*

2 cups dark grape juice
¾ cup coconut cream
¼-½ cup tahini
2 tablespoons carob powder
1 teaspoon vanilla

Blend all ingredients at high speed. Pour into a container and freeze.
    Serve with chopped fresh fruit.

Vanilla Icecream

Free of dairy products, wheat, yeast, corn, sugar, eggs, soy, orange and nightshades.　　*Serves 3-4*

4 small bananas, peeled, chopped and
**   frozen**
½ cup soy milk or thick nut milk
1 teaspoon vanilla
1 tablespoon tahini
½-1 tablespoon honey

Blend ingredients and freeze.
    Serve with fruit.

Tropical Freeze

Free of dairy products, wheat, yeast, corn, sugar, eggs, soy, orange and nightshades.　　*Serves 4-5*

4 medium bananas
¼ pawpaw
1 slice pineapple
¾ cup coconut cream or yoghurt
3 passionfruit

Blend all ingredients except passionfruit. Stir in passionfruit and freeze.

Banana-Apricot Sherbet

Free of dairy products, wheat, yeast, corn, sugar, eggs, soy, orange and nightshades. *Serves 4*

Sufficient fresh apricots or peaches, or soaked dried apricots or peaches to provide 2 cups puree when blended
2 medium bananas
1 cup orange or apple juice
½ cup nut butter or natural yoghurt

Blend all ingredients and pour into 1 large or 2 small trays. Freeze until edges harden. Blend again until smooth and fluffy. Return to trays and freeze.
Serve with fresh fruit.

Strawberry Sorbet

Free of dairy products, wheat, yeast, corn, sugar, eggs, soy, orange and nightshades. *Serves 4*

2 punnets strawberries (500 g)
½ cup apple juice
½ cup water
¼ cup honey or maple syrup

Blend all ingredients. Freeze in separate small containers such as icy pole moulds. Before serving, remove from freezer and allow to soften sufficiently to permit blending. Blend and pour icy mixture into open champagne glasses or dishes and top with a whole strawberry and/or grated unsweetened carob.

Plum Pudding

Free of dairy products, wheat, corn, sugar, eggs, soy, orange and nightshades. *Serves 8*

250 g sultanas
250 g chopped raisins
250 g chopped dates
½ cup mixed peel
½ cup chopped almonds
6 tablespoons brandy
rind and juice 1 lemon
1 ½ cups water or apple juice
3 tablespoons agar* flakes
½ cup chopped dried apricots
1 large apple, peeled and grated
1 ½ cups ground sunflower seeds
1 ¼ cups organic millet meal
1 teaspoon cinnamon
½ teaspoon nutmeg
½ teaspoon ground ginger
½ teaspoon mixed spice
½ teaspoon bicarb soda

Combine sultanas, raisins, dates, mixed peel, almonds, brandy, rind and lemon juice. Soak overnight or as long as desired. Combine apple juice, agar flakes and apricots and leave to stand overnight in a pan. Add remaining ingredients to soaked fruit mixture, combining well. Heat apple/agar mixture and simmer till agar has dissolved. Mash the apricots a little. Add apple/agar mixture to fruit mixture, stirring all ingredients well together. Place into a lightly greased pudding basin. Cover top of basin with greaseproof paper, and then foil. Pour 2 cups water into a crockpot and cook pudding on high for 8 hours. Alternatively half fill large saucepan (a jam-making one would be suitable), bring water to boil, lower basin into water and simmer for 4-6 hours.
Serve with brandy custard.
*See note on agar in Glossary.

Brandy Custard

Free of dairy products, wheat, corn, sugar, eggs, soy, orange and nightshades.

3 cups pleasant tasting soy or thick nut milk
1-3 tablespoons honey
1 teaspoon vanilla
3 tablespoons kuzu mixed in 3 tablespoons water, or 4 ½ tablespoons cornflour, mixed in a little water
6 tablespoons brandy

Heat soy or nut milk gently until very hot. Add honey and vanilla and stir well. Add kuzu or cornflour paste and stir till mixture thickens. Remove from heat and add brandy.

Layered Fruit Salad

Free of dairy products, wheat, corn, sugar, eggs, soy, orange and nightshades.   *Serves 8*

2 cups chopped pawpaw
2 cups chopped apple
2 cups purple grapes
3 kiwi fruit, peeled and sliced
3 mandarins, peeled and separated into segments
1 punnet strawberries washed and hulled, then halved

In an attractive glass dish, arrange fruit in layers, beginning with pawpaw.

Serve with cashew cream or tahini cream.

Incredibly Easy Pie

Free of dairy products, wheat, yeast, corn, sugar, soy, orange and nightshades.   *Serves 4*

3 eggs
½ cup brown rice flour or barley flour
2 cups pleasant tasting liquid soy milk or thick nut milk
¼- ½ cup honey
1 cup coconut
2 teaspoons vanilla

Blend all ingredients. Pour into greased pie plate. Bake in moderate oven ½-¾ hour or until set.

Serve with stewed fruit.

Variation

Chop 2 apples finely and place on bottom of plate. Sprinkle with cinnamon before pouring the mixture on top.

Orange Slice

Free of dairy products, wheat, yeast, corn, sugar, eggs, soy and nightshades.   *Serves 4-6*

Base

Nutty rice crust, baked

Filling

2 tablespoons agar* flakes
⅔ cup orange juice
**1 cup pleasant tasting liquid soy milk or
   thick nut milk**
½ teaspoon orange essence
2 teaspoons orange rind
⅓ cup honey

Soak agar in orange juice. Blend together milk, orange essence, orange rind and honey. Bring orange juice and agar to boil, continue to simmer until agar is dissolved. Blend with other ingredients and immediately pour over pie crust. Refrigerate.

Topping

1 cup orange juice
1 tablespoon honey
3 teaspoons agar
pulp 2 passionfruit

Mix agar, orange juice, passionfruit and honey together, and cook as before. Allow to cool and begin to set. Spoon over filling when set and refrigerate.

* See note on agar in Glossary.

Pears in Grape Juice

Free of dairy products, wheat, corn, sugar, eggs, soy, orange and nightshades.   *Serves 5-6*

6-8 pears
3 cups dark grape juice
1 stick cinnamon
1 strip lemon rind

Carefully peel pears leaving stalk intact, keeping pear as even as possible. Pour juice into a saucepan and add cinnamon and lemon rind. Stand pears in juice and gently poach until just tender. From time to time spoon the liquid over the pears. If a deeper colour is desired, add a few drops beetroot juice (this will not affect the taste, only the colour). When tender, chill pears and juice before serving.

Serve with carob sauce (see Sauces section).

Strawberry Jelly

Free of dairy products, wheat, yeast, corn, sugar, eggs, soy, orange and nightshades.   *Serves 6*

2 tablespoons agar* flakes
1 cup water
2 punnets (500 g) strawberries
1 cup apple juice
¼-½ cup honey

Soak agar in water overnight or for 1-2 hours. Heat agar and water until boiling and simmer until flakes dissolve. Blend strawberries, juice and honey. Combine strawberry mixture with agar and blend briefly. Pour into a mould and refrigerate until set.

Serve with fresh strawberries and nut cream, tahini cream or tofu cream.

* See note on agar in Glossary.

Fruit Jelly

Free of dairy products, wheat, yeast, corn, sugar, eggs, soy, orange and nightshades.   *Serves 6*

**2 tablespoons agar* flakes, soaked in
½ cup water and ½ cup fruit juice**
3 cups unsweetened fruit juice
3 cups finely chopped fresh fruit

Bring agar mixture to boil and simmer till flakes have dissolved. Add to remaining fruit juice, mixing well. Stir in fruit. Pour into a mould and refrigerate until set.

   Serve with tahini cream or nut cream.
   *See note on agar in Glossary.

Carob Dessert Cake

**Free of dairy products, wheat, corn, sugar, orange and nightshades.
Can be free of eggs.**   *Serves 4-6*

125 g tofu
¼ cup carob powder
¾ cup pear juice
¾ cup brown rice flour
1 teaspoon cream of tartar
1 teaspoon bicarbonate of soda
½ teaspoon pure vanilla
2-3 tablespoons honey
2 egg whites, with pinch of cream of tartar*

Blend all ingredients except egg whites. Beat egg whites until stiff and fold into mixture. Spoon into lightly greased cake tin and bake 30 minutes in moderate oven.

Note: If tofu is dry and crumbly more pear juice may need to be added.

   * This cake can be made without the egg whites following the above method. However, it will be heavier and will not rise as well.

Carob Topping

¼ cup light carob powder
¼ cup water
1 tablespoon tahini
1-2 teaspoons honey

Simmer carob and water, stirring well until smooth and thick. Stir in tahini and honey. Remove from heat, cool and spread over cake. Decorate cake with coconut or nuts.

With Carob Custard and Berry Filling

**Free of dairy products, wheat, yeast, sugar, eggs, soy, orange and nightshades.
Can be made free of corn by omitting cornflour.**

Carob Custard

¾ cup carob soy milk or thick nut milk
2 tablespoons maple syrup or honey
1 teaspoon vanilla
**1 tablespoon kuzu or 1½ tablespoons
   cornflour mixed with 2 tablespoons
   water**

Make cake several hours or night before. Cut in half.
   Combine all ingredients except kuzu in a saucepan. Heat gently and mix in kuzu or cornflour. Stir until thickened. Spread berry jam (see Spread Section) to thickness desired over bottom half of cake. Cover with a layer of carob custard. Place top half of cake over custard and spread with carob topping.

Baked Apples

Free of dairy, wheat, corn, sugar, eggs, soy, orange and nightshades.

Granny Smith apples, as many as required **finely chopped nuts and raisins** **cinnamon**	Remove core from apples. Fill hollow with nuts and raisins. Dust with cinnamon. Bake for 30 minutes. Serve with yoghurt, nut cream or tofu cream.

Creme Caramel

Free of dairy products, wheat, yeast, corn, sugar, soy, eggs, orange and nightshades.   *Serves 5*

1 ½ tablespoons agar* flakes
5 tablespoons maple syrup
2 cups coconut milk
2 cups pleasant tasting liquid soy milk or
**   thick nut milk**
2 tablespoons honey
3-4 teaspoons vanilla
	Soak agar flakes overnight or for 1-2 hours in 1 cup of coconut milk. Lightly grease 5 individual moulds for example souffle dishes. Pour 1 tablespoon maple syrup into each dish and rotate so as to coat base and sides with syrup. Bring agar mixture to the boil, then simmer until dissolved. Stir in the remaining coconut milk, soy milk, honey and vanilla. Blend well till smooth and pour into moulds straight away. Refrigerate until set. Run a knife around inside edge of moulds to loosen custard. Invert onto a plate.
	    Serve with nut cream.
	    * See note on agar in Glossary.

Lemon Curd Pie

Free of dairy products, wheat, yeast, corn, sugar, soy, orange and nightshades.   *Serves 4-5*

Base

Millet/coconut crust

Filling

3 eggs **½ cup lemon juice** **2 ½ tablespoons honey** **rind 1 lemon** **2 apples, peeled and grated** **cinnamon**	Blend eggs, juice, honey and rind. Pour into pie shell and sprinkle with apple. Dust with a little cinnamon. Bake in a moderate oven for approximately 30 minutes.

Mango Yoghurt Pie

Free of wheat, corn, sugar, eggs, orange and nightshades. Can be made free of dairy products if yoghurt is omitted. Can be made free of soy if tofu is omitted.   *Serves 6*

Base

Coconut/nut crust, baked

Filling

2½ tablespoons agar* flakes
1 cup apple or orange juice
1½ cups (2 large) chopped mangoes
400 g non-fat yoghurt or 200 g blended tofu
1-2 tablespoons maple syrup or honey
**   (optional)**

Soak agar overnight or 1-2 hours in juice. Heat until flakes have dissolved. Blend mango. Pour mango puree into agar mixture, stirring well. Stir in yoghurt or tofu and maple syrup, mixing thoroughly. Pour into pie crust and refrigerate until well set.

Topping

3 teaspoons agar* flakes
½ cup apple juice
¾ cup mango puree
pulp 2-3 passionfruit

Soak agar flakes in apple juice. Bring to boil and simmer till well dissolved. Stir in the mango puree and the passionfruit pulp. Spoon over the top of the pie and refrigerate.

Serve with fresh mango slices.

* See note on agar in Glossary.

Baked Banana and Rice Pudding

Free of dairy products, wheat, yeast, corn, sugar, eggs, soy, orange and nightshades.   *Serves 4-5*

1 cup uncooked brown rice
1 cup mashed banana
3 cups nut milk
few drops pure vanilla
rind 1 lemon
1 teaspoon nutmeg

Place all ingredients in casserole dish except nutmeg. Stir well. Sprinkle nutmeg over top, using a tea strainer to shake evenly. Bake 1½-2 hours in moderate oven.

Serve with stewed fruit.

Lemon Sauce Pudding

Free of dairy products, wheat, yeast, corn, sugar, orange, soy and nightshades.   *Serves 4*

¼-½ **cup honey**
½ **cup lemon juice**
rind 1 lemon
2 cups pleasant tasting soy milk or
   coconut cream
1 teaspoon vanilla
4 tablespoons brown rice flour
½ **teaspoon bicarbonate of soda**
1 teaspoon cream of tartar
4 eggs, separated

Mix together or blend all ingredients except egg whites. Beat egg whites till stiff and fold into mixture. Lightly grease a casserole dish and pour in pudding mixture. Stand in shallow pan of water and bake in moderate oven approximately 30-40 minutes. Serve with tahini cream.

Rhubarb Fool with Tofu Lemon Cream

Free of dairy products, wheat, yeast, corn, sugar, eggs, soy, orange and nightshades.   *Serves 6*

4 medium to large cooking apples
1 bunch rhubarb

Slice apples finely and chop stalks of rhubarb. Poach with a little water and honey to taste. Refrigerate until cold.

Tofu Lemon Cream

Free of dairy products, wheat, corn, sugar, eggs, orange and nightshades.

400 g tofu
½ **cup lemon juice**
grated rind of 2 lemons
maple syrup to taste

Blend tofu, lemon juice, rind and maple syrup. Layer rhubarb mixture and cream in tall glasses. Approximately ⅔ cup rhubarb to ⅓ cup cream or more per glass, finishing with cream. Top with cinnamon, grated unsweetened carob or a pecan nut. Serve well chilled.

Note: This will keep well overnight.

Lemon Tarts

Free of dairy products, wheat, yeast, sugar, soy, eggs, corn, orange and nightshades.   *Makes 18*

1 quantity nutty rice crust — see Dessert
   section
1 quantity lemon topping using variation —
   see Spread section — for these tarts
   use apple juice instead of water
cashew cream or ricotta cream to garnish
   — see Dessert section and Icing section
   respectively

Press crust mixture into lightly greased shallow patty trays. Bake in a moderate oven until cooked. Leave to cool. Just before tarts are to be served, fill with lemon topping. Spoon a dollop of cashew cream or ricotta cream onto filling.

Strawberry Tarts

Free of dairy products, wheat, yeast, soy, sugar, eggs, corn, orange and nightshades.　　*Makes 18*

**1 quantity of nutty rice crust (see Dessert
　section)**
**½ quantity strawberry topping (see
　Spreads)**
½ punnet strawberries extra

Press crust mixture into lightly-greased shallow patty trays. Bake in moderate oven until cooked. Leave to cool.

Just before tarts are to be served fill with strawberry topping. Place a strawberry in the centre of each tart.

Strawberry Sponge Shortcake

Free of dairy products, wheat, yeast, soy, sugar, corn, orange and nightshades.　　*Serves 6*

Crust

**1 quantity gingerbread cookie mixture but
　omit ginger and carob and substitute
　1 teaspoon vanilla
　4-5 tablespoons natural berry jam**

Sponge

½ quantity of sponge cake mix

Strawberry Topping

**½ quantity of topping (see recipe in
　Spreads section)**
1 punnet strawberries — hulled

Make up cookie mixture and press into a lightly-greased pie dish. Bake in a moderate oven until lightly browned. Remove and cool. Make up sponge according to instructions and pour into a lightly-greased pie dish slightly smaller than that used for crust. Bake in moderate oven until firm. Remove and cool.

Make up quantity of strawberry topping and refrigerate until ready for use.

Spread jam over base of pie crust. Turn out sponge and place into pie crust on top of jam. Spread topping over sponge. Top with strawberries.

Carob Mousse

Free of dairy products, wheat, yeast, corn, sugar, eggs, soy, orange and nightshades.　　*Serves 4-6*

1 cup fresh chopped dates
1 ¼ cups nut milk
**⅓ cup cereal coffee powder or instant
　dandelion powder**
⅓ cup carob powder
½ cup tahini
few drops vanilla
1 teaspoon pure orange essence (optional)
2 tablespoons maple syrup
2 teaspoons grated orange rind (optional)
1 teaspoon cinnamon
¼ teaspoon nutmeg
1 cup water
1 heaped tablespoon agar*

Place dates, milk, dandelion or cereal coffee, carob powder, tahini, vanilla, orange essence, maple syrup, orange rind, cinnamon and nutmeg into blender, blend until smooth. Pour water into a saucepan and stir in agar. Cook until agar has dissolved. Quickly place in blender with other ingredients and blend once more. Pour into serving dishes.

Serve with a dollop of cashew cream in the centre of each dish and garnish with a strawberry.

* See note on agar in Glossary.

Fruit Mousse

Free of dairy products, wheat, yeast, corn, sugar, eggs, soy, orange and nightshades.   *Serves 5-6*

3 cups mango and passionfruit pulp (or any other choice of fruit) 1 cup pleasant tasting liquid soy milk or thick nut milk ½ cup water 2 tablespoons agar flakes* ¼ cup lemon juice 1-2 tablespoons honey	Mix fruit pulp and milk in a bowl. Place water, agar flakes, lemon juice and honey into a saucepan. Cook until agar flakes have dissolved. Add agar mixture to fruit pulp and milk. Blend until smooth. Pour into individual glass dishes. Serve chilled and garnished with a strawberry and a sprig of mint. * See note on agar in Glossary. + When using fruit that is not sweet it may be necessary to add 2-4 tablespoons honey or 1-2 bananas.

Tahini Cream

Free of dairy products, wheat, yeast, corn, sugar, eggs, soy, orange and nightshades.

¼ cup tahini ¾ cup pleasant tasting liquid soy milk or thick nut milk 2 teaspoons vanilla ¼ cup honey or maple syrup	Blend all ingredients together and chill. Use as a cream over fruit and pies.

Carob Tahini Cream

As above but add 1 tablespoon carob powder.

Both these creams are delicious and may be either partially frozen before use, or thickened to the consistency of whipped cream.

Thickened Tahini Cream

Free of dairy products, wheat, yeast, corn, sugar, eggs, soy, orange and nightshades.

Use the same ingredients as for tahini cream but add 2 teaspoons agar* flakes.	Heat milk until flakes dissolve. Combine all ingredients. Mix well and refrigerate. * See note on agar in Glossary.

Tofu Cream

Free of dairy products, wheat, corn, sugar, eggs, orange and nightshades.

1 cup mashed tofu (be sure tofu is fresh) 1-3 tablespoons honey 1 teaspoon pure vanilla	Blend ingredients thoroughly. Serve over fresh fruit, pies and jellies.

Ricotta Cream

See recipe for ricotta icing.

Nut Cream

Free of dairy products, wheat, yeast, corn, sugar, eggs, soy, orange and nightshades.

**1 cup cashews, pecans or blanched
    almonds
water to desired consistency
honey to taste**

Blend or grind nuts as finely as possible. Add water gradually until desired consistency is reached. Mix in enough honey to sweeten to taste.
    Serve over pies and fruits.

Custard

Free of dairy products, wheat, yeast, sugar, eggs, soy, orange and nightshades.
Can be free of corn if cornflour is omitted.

**2 cups pleasant tasting liquid soy milk or
    thick nut milk
2 tablespoons kuzu mixed in 2 tablespoons
    water of 3 tablespoons cornflour in
    3 tablespoons water
1 teaspoon-2 tablespoons honey
1-2 teaspoons vanilla**

Heat milk gently until hot. Stir in kuzu or cornflour paste, simmer until mixture thickens. Add honey and vanilla. Cool slightly and serve over desserts.

Note: Best made with kuzu or cornflour not arrowroot.
    Serve hot or cold over stewed fruit.

SAUCES

The addition of a sauce to an ordinary dish can turn it into a gourmet delight. Included in this section are savoury and sweet sauces.

SAVOURY SAUCES

Mushroom Sauce
Free of dairy products, wheat, corn, sugar, eggs, orange and nightshades.

1 cup finely chopped mushrooms
1 cup water
dash tamari
2 teaspoons lemon juice
1 tablespoon arrowroot or kuzu mixed in
   1 tablespoon water
dash freshly ground black pepper
	Place mushrooms and water in a saucepan. Bring to the boil, then add tamari and lemon juice. Add arrowroot or kuzu paste to mushrooms and stir till thickened. Add pepper.
	   Serve over patties, fish, chicken or fritters.

Chinese Sauce
Free of dairy products, wheat, corn, sugar, egg, orange and nightshades.

1 ¼ cups vegetable stock or water **dash tamari** **2 tablespoons sherry or port or mirin** **1-2 garlic cloves, crushed** **2 slices finely chopped ginger** **2 tablespoons kuzu or 1 ½ tablespoons** **arrowroot mixed in 2 tablespoons water**	Mix stock or water, tamari, sherry, garlic and ginger in a small saucepan. Bring mixture to the boil. Add kuzu or arrowroot paste to other ingredients and stir till thickened. Can be served over vegetables.

Plum Pudding (p76) with Brandy Custard (p77)

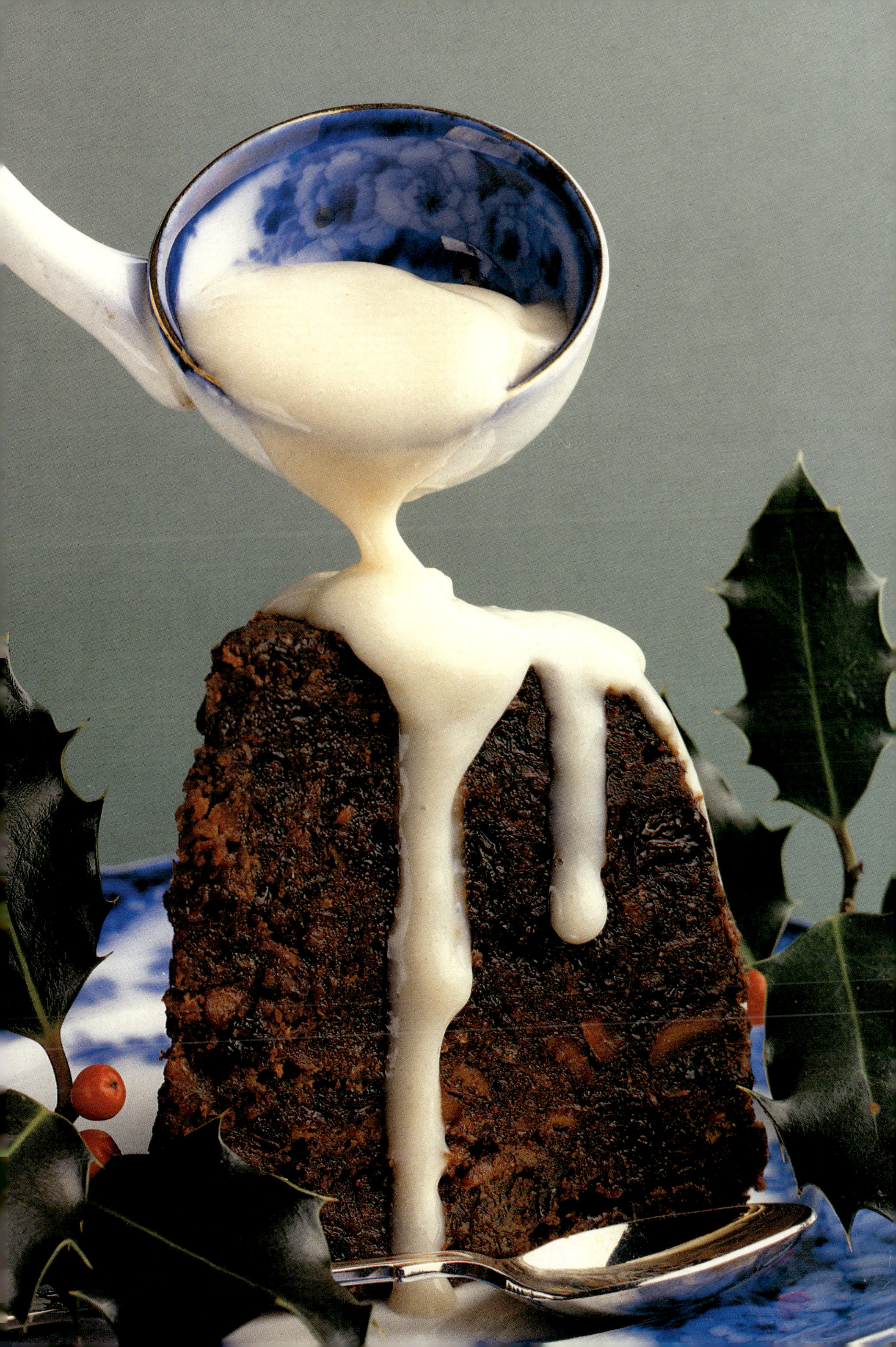

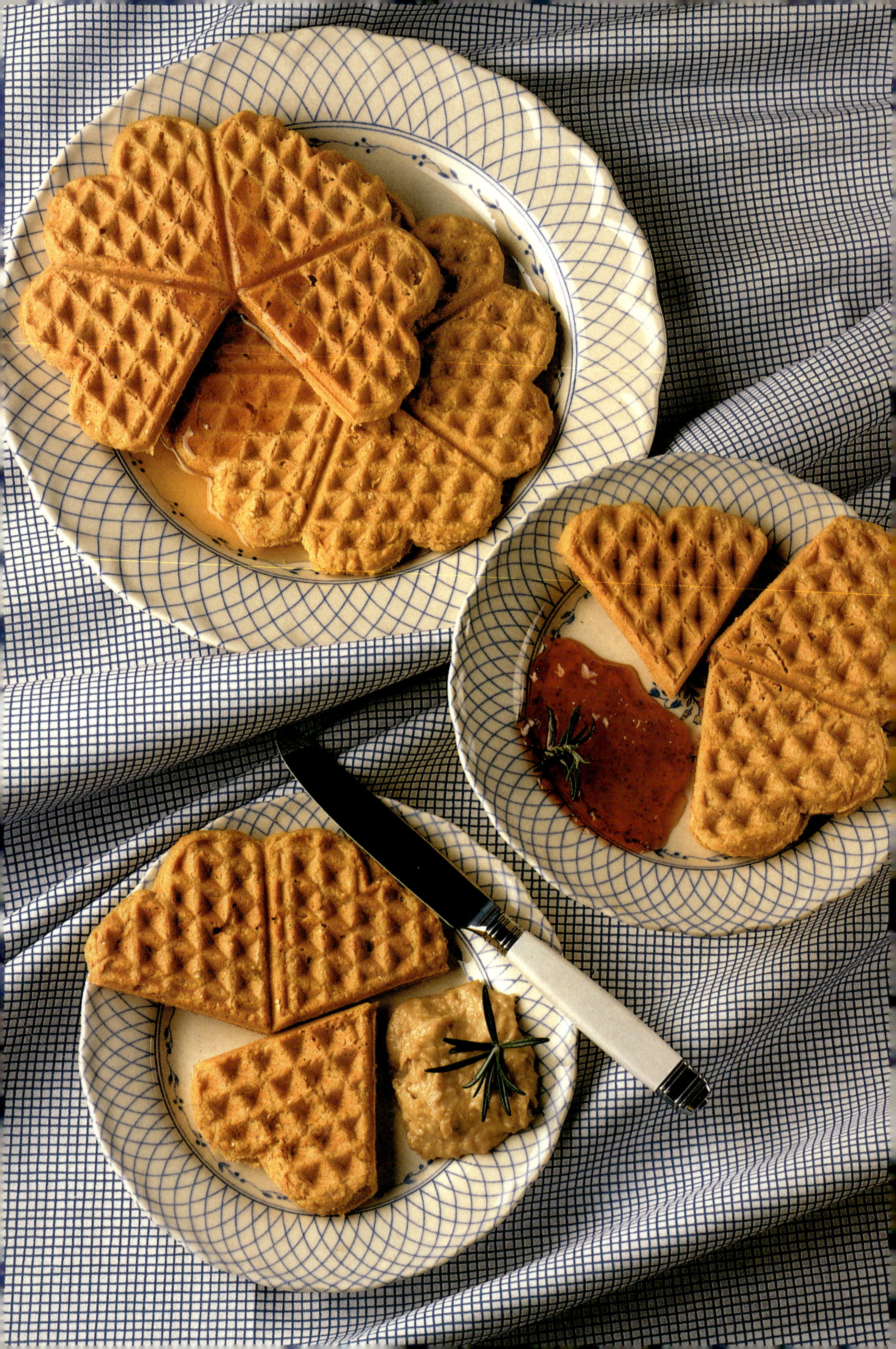

Sweet and Sour Sauce

Free of dairy products, wheat, corn, sugar, eggs, soy and orange.

1 cup pineapple juice 1 tablespoon tomato paste 1 tablespoon apple cider vinegar 1 tablespoon kuzu or arrowroot mixed in 1 tablespoon water	Mix pineapple juice, tomato paste and vinegar in a saucepan. Bring mixture to the boil. Add kuzu or arrowroot paste to juice mixture and stir till thickened. Serve over fish or chicken.

Tomato Sauce

Free of dairy products, wheat, corn, sugar, eggs and orange.
Can be made free of yeast and soy by omitting tamari.

4-5 small tomatoes, chopped finely 1 finely chopped onion 2 cloves garlic, crushed ½ cup apple juice 2 teaspoons tomato paste dash tamari or herbal seasoning ½ teaspoon nutmeg 1/8 teaspoon ground allspice 3 shallots or 1-2 tablespoons finely chopped parsley	Cook all ingredients together, except shallots and parsley, for 20 minutes. Add shallots or parsley before serving. Serve over fish, nut loaves or vegetarian rolls.

Nugget Sauce

Free of dairy products, wheat, yeast, corn, sugar, eggs, soy and orange.
Can be free of nightshades if sweet potato is used.

¾ cup cooked potatoes or kumera 1 medium carrot, cooked ¾-1 cup water 1 tablespoon lemon juice 2 tablespoons cashews or blanched almonds dash herbal seasoning	Blend all ingredients thoroughly and serve over vegetables.

Millet and Pumpkin Waffles (p94) with Strawberry Jam (p102) and Cashew Cream (p85)

Soy White Sauce

Free of dairy products, wheat, corn, sugar, eggs, orange and nightshades.
Can be made free of yeast by omitting tamari.

**1 cup soy milk (ready made and pleasant
    tasting such as Bon Soy)**
**1 tablespoon kuzu or arrowroot mixed in 2
    tablespoons stock or water**
juice ½ lemon
dash tamari or herbal seasoning
**1 tablespoon finely chopped herbs,
    e.g. basil**
freshly ground black pepper

Bring soy milk gently to the boil. Add kuzu or arrowroot paste to milk and stir till mixture thickens. Add remaining ingredients. Garnish with extra herbs or finely chopped red capsicum.

Serve over asparagus or cauliflower.

Coconut White Sauce

Free of dairy products, wheat, yeast, corn, sugar, eggs, soy, orange and nightshades.

2 tablespoons finely chopped celery
1 tablespoon finely chopped onion
2 tablespoons finely chopped parsley
2 tablespoons brown rice flour
1 cup coconut milk
1 tablespoon flaked almonds

Saute celery, onion and parsley. Add flour and stir. Slowly add coconut milk, stirring until thickened. Garnish with the flaked almonds.

Serve over cauliflower.

Spicy Nut Sauce

Free of dairy products, wheat, corn, sugar, eggs and orange.

1 cup chopped onion
2 cloves garlic, crushed
1 bay leaf
2 teaspoons finely chopped ginger
1 tablespoon honey
**1 cup hazelnut butter made from roasted
    hazelnuts**
¼ teaspoon cayenne pepper
juice 1 lemon
1 tablespoon apple cider vinegar
2 cups water
dash tamari or herbal seasoning

Saute onion, garlic, bay leaf and ginger. When onion becomes transparent add remaining ingredients and mix thoroughly. Simmer on very low heat for 20-30 minutes or until mixture is quite thick. Remove bay leaf.

Serve over vegetables or sprouts, either hot or cold.

SWEET SAUCES

Strawberry Sauce (1)

Free of dairy products, wheat, yeast, corn, sugar, eggs, soy, orange and nightshades.

1 250 g punnet strawberries
1 tablespoon honey
¼ cup water or apple juice
1 heaped tablespoon arrowroot or kuzu
     mixed in 2 tablespoons water
	Blend strawberries, honey and water or juice. Place in a saucepan and heat gently. Add arrowroot or kuzu paste to strawberries and stir till thickened.
	     Serve over waffles or pancakes.

Strawberry Sauce (2)

Free of dairy products, wheat, yeast, corn, sugar, eggs, soy, orange and nightshades.

1 250 g punnet strawberries **¼ cup apple juice** **¼ cup water** **¼ cup honey**	Blend ingredients and pour over fruit or icecream.

Apple Sauce

Free of dairy products, wheat, yeast, corn, sugar, eggs, soy, orange and nightshades.

2 juicy apples, peeled and grated **½ cup nut cream** **1 tablespoon honey**	Blend ingredients and pour over fruit, cereal or rice.

Custard Apple Sauce

Free of dairy products, wheat, yeast, corn, sugar, eggs, soy and nightshades.

flesh of 1 large custard apple **juice ½ lemon** **juice 1 orange** **pulp 2 passionfruit**	Blend all ingredients except passionfruit. Add passionfruit and refrigerate. Serve over fruit, icecream or jelly.

Carob Sauce

Free of dairy products, wheat, yeast, corn, sugar, eggs, soy, orange and nightshades.

1 cup nut milk
¼ cup maple syrup
1 tablespoon carob powder
few drops pure vanilla
1 tablespoon arrowroot mixed in
     1 tablespoon water
	Blend nut milk, maple syrup, carob powder and vanilla. Place in saucepan and heat gently. Add arrowroot paste to other ingredients and stir till thickened.
	     Serve hot or cold over fruit.

BREADS

For those allergic to yeast and wheat/gluten, bread may be sorely missed, especially on occasions when a sandwich is quick and easy to prepare and eat. These breads are different from commercial breads in texture and flavour but they are tasty, sustaining and nutritious.

Seed Bread

Free of dairy products, wheat, yeast, corn, sugar, eggs, soy, orange and nightshades.

1 cup soy flour or brown rice flour
1 cup arrowroot flour
½ cup buckwheat flour
1 teaspoon bicarbonate of soda
2 teaspoons cream tartar
½ cup sunflower seeds
¼ cup sesame seeds
¼ cup linseed
¼ cup carraway seeds
1 ¼ - 1 ½ cups nut or soy milk
2 teaspoons honey

Sift flours, cream of tartar and bicarbonate of soda. Add seeds to flours. Mix honey and nut milk together and stir into dry ingredients. Pour into lightly greased loaf tin and bake in moderate oven until bread comes away from tin (approximately 40-45 minutes). Wait until cold before slicing with a sharp knife.

Can be toasted under griller or sliced and returned to oven until crisp.

Millet Buckwheat Bread

Free of dairy products, wheat, yeast, corn, sugar, eggs, orange and nightshades.
Can be free of soy if ground nuts are used.

¾ cup millet meal (rolled millet ground to a meal)
½ cup buckwheat flour
½ cup buckwheat groats
½ cup soy powder or ground nuts
½ teaspoon bicarbonate of soda
1 teaspoon cream tartar
½ teaspoon ground ginger
1 teaspoon cinnamon
¾ cup sunflower seeds
1 ½ cups apple juice or water
2 tablespoons honey

Combine dry ingredients. Add blended apple juice and honey. Pour into lightly greased tray and bake in moderate oven approximately 30-35 minutes or until bread comes away from tin. Wait until cold before cutting into squares.

Slice in half and serve with your choice of spread.

Pumpkin Rice Bread

Free of dairy products, wheat, yeast, corn, sugar, eggs, soy, orange and nightshades.

1 ¼ cups brown rice flour
¾ cup buckwheat flour
3 tablespoons rolled millet
1 teaspoon bicarbonate of soda
2 teaspoons cream of tartar
1 ½ cups almond milk
¼ cup mashed steamed pumpkin or
    apricot puree*
1-2 tablespoons honey

Combine dry ingredients in bowl. Blend liquid ingredients and mix into dry ingredients stirring well. Pour into lightly greased loaf tin and bake in moderate oven (approximately 35-40 minutes) or until bread comes away from tin. Wait until cold before slicing.

    * Apricot puree: 125 g apricots
                1 cup water
Simmer until tender and blend.

Gluten Free Bread

Free of dairy products, wheat, yeast, corn, sugar, soy, orange and nightshades.

1 ¼ cups rice flour
¼ cup millet meal (ground from rolled
    millet)
¼ cup buckwheat flour
1 teaspoon bicarbonate of soda
2 teaspoons cream of tartar
1 teaspoon cinnamon
1 cup grated carrot, firmly packed
3 small bananas, mashed or 1 grated apple
2 eggs or 3 egg whites stiffly beaten
¾ cup soy or nut milk

Combine dry ingredients. Add grated carrot. Blend eggs, milk and bananas (if using egg whites only, fold in last). Combine with dry ingredients mixing well. Pour into a small lightly greased loaf tin and bake in moderate oven (approximately 40-45 minutes). Slice when cold.

Sunflower and Sesame Seed Loaf

Free of dairy products, wheat, yeast, corn, sugar, eggs, soy and nightshades.

¾ cup brown rice flour
½ cup buckwheat flour
1 cup arrowroot flour
1 teaspoon bicarbonate of soda
2 teaspoons cream of tartar
grated rind of 1 orange
½ cup sunflower seeds, ground
¼ cup sesame seeds, ground
¼ cup linseed, ground
2 tablespoons nuts, ground
1 tablespoon honey
1 ¼-1 ½ cups almond or soy milk

Sift flours, bicarbonate soda and cream of tartar together. Add nuts, seeds and rind. Blend honey with milk. Pour into bowl, mixing all ingredients together. Place mixture into lightly greased tin and bake in moderate oven approximately 45 minutes or until cooked. Remove from tin when cooked and allow to cool.

Sprouted Pizza Bread

Free of dairy products, yeast, corn, sugar, eggs, soy and nightshades.

2 cups organic wheat grain
pure water for soaking

Soak wheat overnight. Drain off water and leave to sprout until the sprout is the length of the grain. Rinse and drain only enough to encourage sprouting. Spread the grain out on a tray for an hour or more to dry off any excess moisture. Grind in a blender or a hand grinder or Champion juicer to make a fine dough. Lightly grease 2 baking trays, then press dough onto trays until it becomes very thin, approximately ¼ cm in thickness. (It is best to use a little flour for this as dough is sticky.) Place in a very low oven — about 40 degrees C and leave for 48 hours or until bread is crisp.

Variation:

Add any herbs or spices of choice to the dough.

Waffles, Pancakes, Scones and Muffins

These are a wonderful way to provide children (and adults of course) with wholegrains, providing one answer to the problem of the ubiquitous sandwich and morning toast. In the following recipes a range of grains has been used and those on allergy-free or rotation diets should find one or more to fit the occasion, be it breakfast, lunch or a fine and filling dessert.

Note: If not serving immediately, place on a wire rack to prevent them becoming soggy, or crisp on a rack in a low oven for crunchy biscuits.

Millet Waffles

Free of dairy products, wheat, yeast, corn, sugar, eggs, soy, orange and nightshades.

2 cups rolled millet
½ cup sunflower seeds
2 tablespoons arrowroot
1 cup water

Grind millet and seeds in blender to make a fine meal. Add arrowroot and water and blend again. Pour enough mixture into the waffle iron to make the desired size of waffles. The number of waffles will depend on the size of the waffle iron and the size of the waffles desired.

Serve waffles warm as they tend to become dry when left to cool.

Millet-Rice Waffles

Free of dairy products, wheat, yeast, corn, sugar, eggs, soy, orange and nightshades.

¾ cup millet flour
1 cup brown rice flour
¾ cup soy or nut milk
½ cup water

Mix all ingredients together well. Pour enough mixture into the waffle iron to make the desired size of waffles. Cook until the iron opens easily.

Barley Waffles (1)

Free of dairy products, wheat, yeast, corn, sugar, soy, orange and nightshades.

2 eggs **2 teaspoons honey** **¾ cup soy or nut milk** **½ cup water** **few drops vanilla** **2 cups barley flour** **½ teaspoon bicarbonate of soda** **1 teaspoon cream of tartar**	Separate eggs. Beat egg yolks, honey, milk, water and vanilla. Sift dry ingredients. Add liquid to dry ingredients and mix well. Beat egg whites until stiff and fold into mixture. Spoon desired amount into hot waffle iron and cook till brown and crisp. Serve with your favourite berry jam or stewed apple.

Barley Waffles (2)

Free of dairy products, wheat, yeast, corn, sugar, eggs, soy, orange and nightshades.

2 cups barley flour **½ teaspoon bicarbonate of soda** **1 teaspoon cream of tartar** **2 cups soy or nut milk or water**	Sift dry ingredients. Add liquid, stirring well. Pour enough mixture into waffle iron to make the desired size of waffles and cook till iron opens easily.

Millet and Pumpkin Waffles

Free of dairy products, wheat, yeast, corn, sugar, soy, orange and nightshades.

½ cup mashed steamed pumpkin **1 cup nut milk** **1 egg, beaten** **2 cups very fine millet meal** **2 tablespoons arrowroot** **2 teaspoons mixed spice**	Combine pumpkin, milk and egg. Add sifted dry ingredients and mix well. Pour enough mixture into waffle iron to make the desired size of waffles. Cook until iron opens easily.

Rice Waffles

Free of dairy products, wheat, yeast, corn, sugar, soy, orange and nightshades. Can be free of egg.

1 ½ cups brown rice flour **¼ teaspoon bicarb soda** **½ teaspoon cream of tartar** **1 cup plus 1 tablespoon nut milk** **1 beaten egg, or omit egg and increase nut milk to 1 ¼ cups**	Sift dry ingredients. Beat nut milk and egg together and stir well into dry ingredients. Pour enough mixture into waffle iron to make the desired size waffles and leave till iron opens easily.

Corn Waffles

Free of dairy products, wheat, yeast, sugar, soy, orange and nightshades.

2 eggs **¾ cup soy or nut milk** **½ cup water** **2 cups barley flour** **½ teaspoon bicarb soda** **1 teaspoon cream of tartar** **2 tablespoons chopped nuts** **2 cooked cobs of corn** **1 finely chopped onion**	Beat eggs, milk and water together. Sift dry ingredients, then add chopped nuts. Add liquid to dry ingredients and mix well. Remove corn from cob. Add corn and finely chopped onion to mixture and stir well. Spoon enough mixture into waffle iron to make the desired size of waffles and cook till iron opens easily.

Sesame Rice Waffles

Free of dairy products, wheat, yeast, corn, sugar, eggs, soy, orange and nightshades.

¾ cup unhulled sesame seeds **1-1¼ cups brown rice flour or** 　**1½ cups millet meal** **3 tablespoons arrowroot** **1½ cups water**	Grind seeds to a fine meal. Add remaining ingredients and blend or mix thoroughly. Pour enough mixture into waffle iron to make the desired size waffles, and leave until iron opens easily.

Banana Pancakes

Free of dairy products, wheat, yeast, corn, sugar, soy, orange and nightshades.

¼ cup arrowroot **¾ cup brown rice flour or millet meal** **¼ teaspoon bicarb soda** **1 teaspoon cream of tartar** **½ teaspoon cinnamon** **½ cup soy or nut milk** **1 teaspoon lemon juice** **1 banana, mashed** **1 beaten egg or 2 stiffly beaten egg whites**	Mix dry ingredients together. Combine milk, lemon juice, mashed banana and beaten egg together, mixing well. If using egg whites, fold in last. Add to dry ingredients, mixing well. Leave to stand 15 minutes. Stir, then pour desired amount of mixture into pan and cook well one side. Turn pancake and briefly cook the other side.

Buckwheat Pancakes (1)

Free of dairy products, wheat, yeast, corn, sugar, eggs, soy, orange and nightshades.

½ cup ground almonds **½ cup buckwheat flour** **¾ cup water**	Blend ingredients thoroughly until smooth. Heat pan and use a small amount of ghee for cooking. Pour desired amount of mixture into pan and cook well one side. Turn pancake and briefly cook the other side.

Buckwheat Pancakes (2)

Free of dairy products, wheat, yeast, corn, sugar, eggs, soy, orange and nightshades.

1 cup buckwheat flour
1 cup water
1 tablespoon arrowroot

Mix ingredients well together. Heat pan and use a small amount of ghee for cooking. Pour desired amount of mixture into pan and cook until the edges of the pancake begin to lift from the pan. Turn pancake and briefly cook the other side.

SCONES AND MUFFINS

Scones and muffins make very satisfying and sustaining snacks for morning and afternoon teas or for children to take to school.

Barley-Rice Pumpkin Scones

Free of dairy products, wheat, yeast, corn, sugar, eggs, soy, orange and nightshades.   *Makes 10*

1 cup barley flour
1½ cups brown rice flour
1 teaspoon bicarb soda
2 teaspoons cream of tartar
1 teaspoon cinnamon
¼ teaspoon mixed spice
½ cup mashed steamed pumpkin
½-1 cup nut milk
1 tablespoon honey

Sift dry ingredients. Blend pumpkin, milk and honey. Combine all ingredients mixing well. Shape into scones and place on a lightly greased tray. Bake in a hot oven for 12 minutes or until cooked.

Sultana Scones

Makes 10

Free of dairy products, wheat, corn, sugar, orange and nightshades.
Can be made free of yeast if sultanas are omitted.

1 cup soy flour
1 cup brown rice flour
1 teaspoon bicarb soda
2 teaspoons cream of tartar
¼ cup sultanas or ¼ cup mashed banana
¾ cup soy milk or nut milk
1 tablespoon honey
1 beaten egg or 2 stiffly beaten egg whites

Sift dry ingredients and add sultanas. Blend milk, honey, banana and egg, and stir into dry ingredients, or omit egg and add egg whites last. Drop tablespoonfuls onto a lightly greased tray and bake in a moderate oven until lightly browned.

Date Scones

Free of dairy products, wheat, yeast, corn, sugar, eggs, soy, orange and nightshades.   *Makes 12*

1 ½ **cups brown rice flour**
½ **cup buckwheat flour**
1 **teaspoon bicarb soda**
2 **teaspoons cream of tartar**
¾ **cup chopped fresh dates**
¾-1 **cup nut milk**
½ **cup stewed apple**

Sift dry ingredients. Add dates, milk and stewed apple, mixing well. Drop by tablespoonfuls on to a lightly greased tray and bake in a moderate oven until lightly browned.

Fruit Muffins

Free of dairy products, wheat, corn, sugar, eggs, soy, orange and nightshades.   *Makes 10-12*

1 ½ **cups barley flour**
½ **cup brown rice flour**
1 **teaspoon bicarb soda**
2 **teaspoons cream of tartar**
½ **cup coconut**
½ **cup chopped raisins**
½ **cup chopped dried apricots**
1 **apple, peeled and grated**
½-⅔ **cup orange juice or nut milk**
1 **cup mashed banana**

Sift flours, bicarb soda and cream of tartar. Add coconut, raisins, apricots and apple, mixing well. Combine juice and banana and add to flour mixture. Spoon into a lightly greased muffin tray. Bake in a moderate oven approximately 20 minutes or until cooked.

Golden Muffins

Free of dairy products, wheat, yeast, corn, sugar, soy, eggs, orange and nightshades.   *Makes 10-12*

2 **cups brown rice flour**
½ **cup millet flour**
1 **teaspoon bicarb soda**
2 **teaspoons cream of tartar**
1 **cup ground almonds**
2 **cups mashed steamed pumpkin**
¼-½ **cup honey**
1-2 **tablespoons nut milk**

Sift flours, bicarb soda and cream of tartar. Add nuts. Blend pumpkin, honey and milk and add to dry ingredients. Spoon into a lightly greased muffin tray and bake in a moderate oven approximately 30 minutes.

Millet Muffins

Free of dairy products, wheat, yeast, corn, sugar, eggs, soy, orange and nightshades.　　*Makes 9*

**2 cups millet flour — finely ground and
　very fresh**
½ cup rolled millet
½ teaspoon bicarb soda
1 teaspoon cream of tartar
1 medium–large apple, peeled and grated
**1 ¼-1 ½ cups nut milk (the finer the flour the
　more liquid will be needed)**
**1-2 tablespoons honey or maple syrup
　(optional)**

Mix the first five ingredients well together. Add nut milk and honey, mixing all well together. Spoon into a lightly greased muffin tray and bake in a moderate oven till firm to touch in the centre. Spread with homemade jam or cashew cream.

Buckwheat Muffins

Free of dairy products, wheat, yeast, corn, sugar, eggs, soy, orange and nightshades.　　*Makes 10*

**1 quantity buckwheat cake mixture (see
Cakes section)**

Spoon into muffin tray and bake in a moderate oven until firm to touch in the centre.

SPREADS

This section provides an excellent range of spreads, both savoury and sweet which are ideal for breads, waffles, crackers and muffins.

SAVOURY SPREADS

Fish Spread

Free of dairy products, wheat, corn, sugar, eggs, soy, orange and nightshades.
Can be free of yeast if apple cider vinegar is omitted.

400 g fresh sardines, gutted ⅓ **cup lemon juice** ½ **tablespoon chopped chives or** ½ **grated onion** ½ **teaspoon mixed herbs** ½ **teaspoon apple cider vinegar (optional)** **1 tablespoon Olive Mayonnaise (optional)** **— see recipe in Dressings section.**	Steam or poach sardines till tender. Allow to cool then remove heads and spine with bones attached. Place all ingredients into a bowl and blend or mash together. Chill.

Chicken Spread

Free of dairy products, wheat, corn, sugar, eggs, orange and nightshades.
Can be made free of yeast and soy if tamari is omitted.

1 cup chopped cooked chicken ¼ **cup chicken or vegetable stock** **1 spring onion, finely chopped** ¼ **cup finely chopped celery** **1-2 teaspoons finely chopped fresh sage** **2 teaspoons lemon juice** **dash tamari or herbal seasoning (optional)**	Blend chicken with stock till smooth. Mix with remaining ingredients.

Tofu Cottage Cheese

Free of dairy products, wheat, corn, sugar, eggs, orange and nightshades.

2 cups mashed tofu **½ cup chopped chives** **1 cup chopped parsley** **2 tablespoons finely minced spring onion** **3 tablespoons apple cider vinegar** **¼ cup lemon juice** **2 teaspoons honey**	Mix together tofu, chives, parsley and onion. Blend cider vinegar, lemon juice and honey and pour over tofu mixture, stirring well.

Savoury Tofu Spread

Free of dairy products, wheat, corn, sugar, eggs and orange.

200 g tofu
1 cup mashed cooked pumpkin
1 tablespoon tamari
1 tablespoon lemon juice
½-1 teaspoon apple cider vinegar
½ teaspoon finely chopped fresh basil
1-2 cloves crushed garlic
1 small onion or spring onion or
   2 tablespoons chopped shallots
   or chives
1 small tomato
1 cup ground sesame seeds
	Blend all ingredients.

Nut Butters

To make nut butter grind ½-1 cup nuts in blender until there is a fine meal. Some nuts, for example cashews and pecans can be ground easily to make a fine paste. Others, e.g. almonds, will need a little water added. How well the nuts are ground will depend on the type of blender or food processor you have.

Hummus, Avocado Dip and Curried Tofu Dip — see Hors d'oeuvres section.

SWEET SPREADS

Apple-Date Spread

Free of dairy products, wheat, yeast, corn, sugar, eggs, soy, orange and nightshades.

1 apple, peeled and cored **6 fresh dates, chopped** **½ cup apple juice**	Blend thoroughly till smooth.

Cashew-Apple Spread

Free of dairy products, wheat, yeast, corn, sugar, eggs, soy, orange and nightshades.

½ cup cashews **1 apple, peeled and cored**	Blend cashews to a fine meal. Add apple, blending until mixture is creamy. **Variation:** Omit apple and substitute 1 banana and ¼ cup orange juice.

Strawberry Topping

Free of dairy products, wheat, yeast, corn, sugar, eggs, soy, orange and nightshades.

1½-2 tablespoons agar* flakes **⅓ cup apple juice** **2 teaspoons lemon juice** **2 tablespoons honey** **1 cup strawberry pulp** **½ cup nut milk or ready-made liquid** ** soy milk**	Soak agar flakes in the apple juice, lemon juice and honey. Cook about 3-5 minutes until agar has dissolved. Blend strawberry pulp and milk and add to agar mixture. Allow to set in fridge. * See note on agar in Glossary.

Lemon Topping

Free of dairy products, wheat, yeast, corn, sugar, eggs, soy, orange and nightshades.

1½ tablespoons agar* flakes **½ cup lemon juice** **¼ cup water or apple juice** **⅓ cup honey** **1 teaspoon lemon rind** **½ cup ready-made liquid soy milk or thick** ** nut milk**	Soak agar in lemon juice, honey and water. Bring to the boil, then simmer till dissolved, approximately 5 minutes. Add lemon rind and milk. Cool, then refrigerate. **Variation:** Add 1 tablespoon kuzu or arrowroot or cornflour mixed with the milk and simmer till thickened a little to give the texture of lemon butter. * See note on agar in Glossary.

Banana-Tahini Spread

Free of dairy products, wheat, yeast, corn, sugar, eggs, soy, orange and nightshades.

1 large banana **1 tablespoon tahini** **lemon juice to taste**	Mash or blend.

Tomato and Passionfruit Jam

Free of dairy products, wheat, yeast, corn, sugar, soy, eggs and orange.

2 cups tomato pulp **2 apples, peeled and chopped** **½-1 cup honey (optional, depending on the sweetness of the fruit)** **1-2 tablespoons agar* flakes** **pulp 8 passionfruit**	Combine tomato pulp, apple and honey in a saucepan and simmer until apple is soft. Blend or mash ingredients. Stir in agar and cook approximately 5 minutes. Add passionfruit. Pour into a clean jar and refrigerate. * See note on agar in glossary.

Berry Jam

Free of dairy products, wheat, yeast, corn, sugar, eggs, soy, orange and nightshades.

300 g berries, e.g. blackberries **1½ cups fruit juice (e.g. apple or pineapple) or water** **2 tablespoons agar* flakes** **1-2 tablespoons honey (optional)**	Combine ingredients in a saucepan and simmer till agar has dissolved. Cool a little, then pour into a clean jar and refrigerate. * See note on agar in glossary.

Mandarin Marmalade

Free of dairy products, wheat, yeast, corn, sugar, eggs, soy and nightshades.

3 mandarins with peel intact, chopped finely **1½ cups water** **1 tablespoon agar* flakes** **1 tablespoon honey** **juice ½ orange** **juice ½ lemon**	Combine ingredients in a saucepan and simmer until agar has dissolved. Cool a little, then pour into a clean jar and refrigerate. * See note on agar in glossary.

Date-Seed Spread

Free of dairy products, wheat, yeast, corn, sugar, eggs, soy, orange and nightshades.

1 cup sunflower seeds **½ cup chopped fresh dates** **1-2 tablespoons lemon juice** **cinnamon to taste**	Blend ingredients and use as a spread on waffles or crackers.

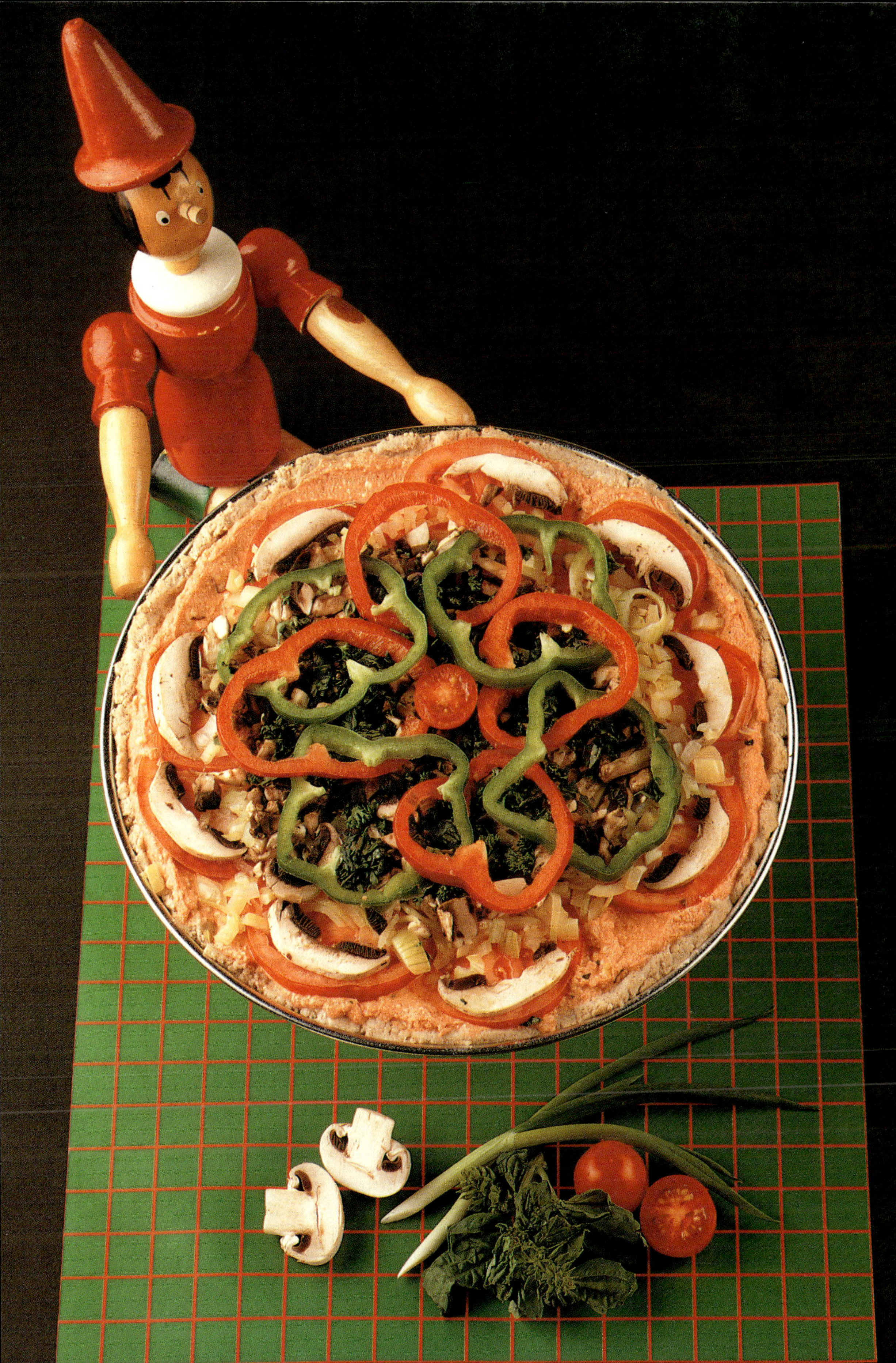

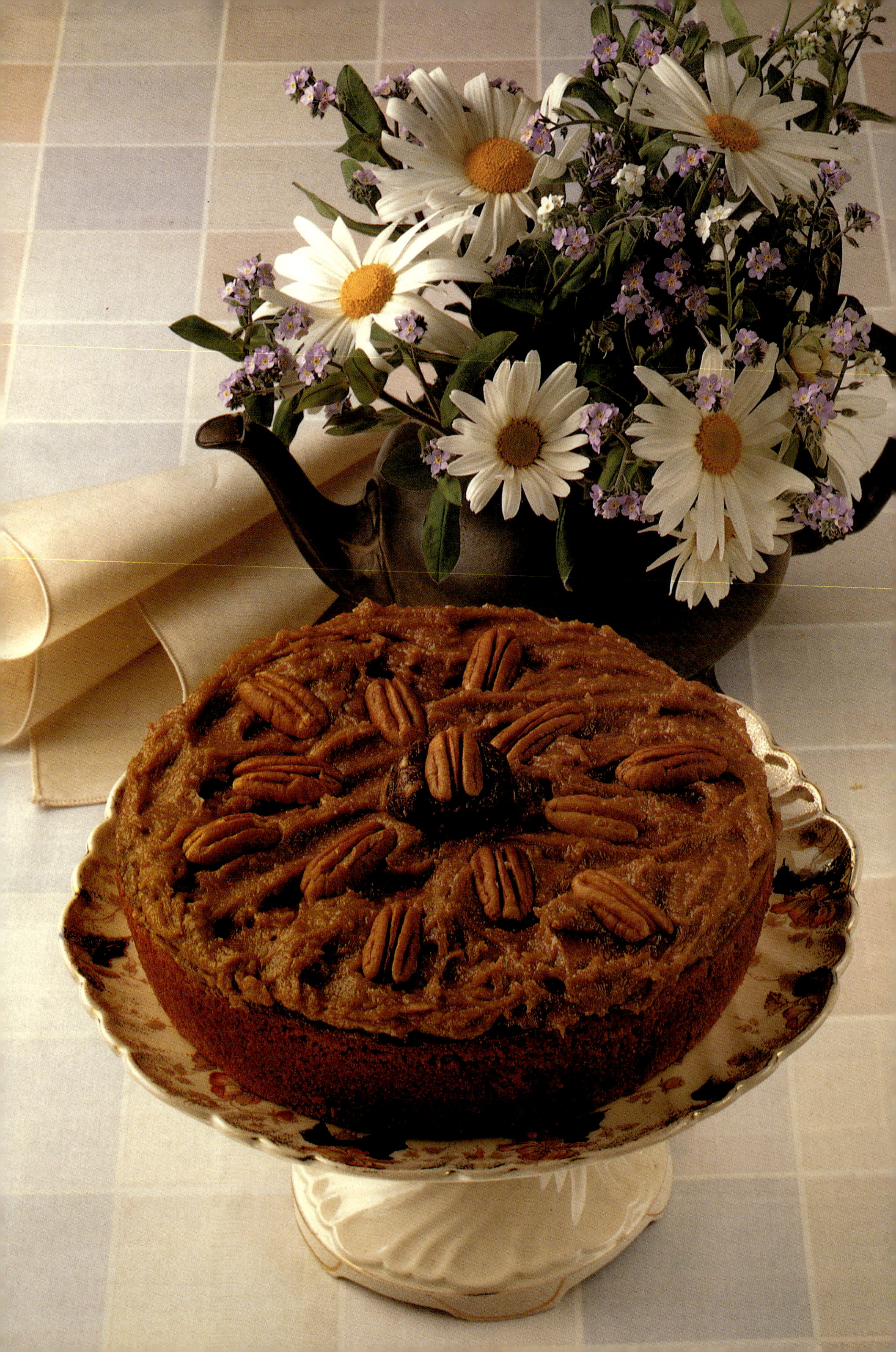

CAKES

These cakes are not really a luxury, but a delicious means of obtaining valuable nutrients. For this reason they can, in moderation, be enjoyed by almost everyone. They are excellent to serve for morning and afternoon teas, and of course are important for celebrations such as birthdays, Christmas and other festive occasions.

Banana Cake (1)

Free of dairy products, wheat, yeast, corn, sugar, eggs, soy, orange and nightshades.

1 cup mashed banana
juice ½ lemon
1 teaspoon bicarb soda
2 teaspoons cream of tartar
⅓ cup tahini
¼-½ cup honey
½ cup soy milk or nut milk
½ cup rolled millet
¼ cup coconut
1 cup brown rice flour
½ cup ground sunflower seeds

Mix together banana, lemon juice, bicarb soda and cream of tartar. Blend tahini, honey and milk and add to banana mixture. Add rolled millet, coconut, brown rice flour and ground sunflower seeds, mixing all ingredients well together. Pour into a lightly greased loaf tin and bake in a moderate oven 40-50 minutes.

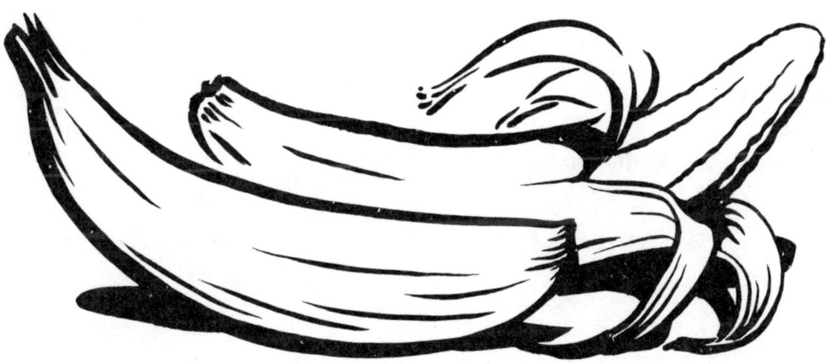

Pizza (p68) ready to go into the oven

Peanut Butter Cake (p109) with 'coffee' icing (p111)

Banana Cake (2)

Free of dairy products, wheat, corn, sugar, soy, orange and nightshades.
Can be made free of yeast by omitting rum.

---

1 ½ **cups barley flour or brown rice flour**
1 ½ **teaspoons bicarb soda**
1 ½ **teaspoons cream of tartar**
½ **cup coconut**
1 **cup mashed banana**
½ **cup nut or soy milk**
1 **teaspoon vanilla**
¼- ½ **cup honey**
1 **beaten egg or 2 stiffly beaten egg whites**

Syrup

1 **tablespoon honey**
2 **tablespoons lemon juice**
1 **tablespoon hot water**
1 **teaspoon rum (optional)**

Sift flour, bicarb soda and cream of tartar. Blend remaining ingredients and combine with flour mixture. If using egg whites only, fold in last. Pour into a lightly greased loaf tin and bake in a moderate oven or until cooked. To make syrup, melt honey in hot water, then add lemon juice and rum. When cake has been removed from the tin, pour half of the syrup mixture over the top of the cake.

Turn cake over and pour remainder of syrup over the bottom.

Carob Cake

Free of dairy products, wheat, yeast, corn, sugar, soy and nightshades.

---

2 **tablespoons carob powder**
1 ½ **cups barley flour**
1 **teaspoon bicarb soda**
2 **teaspoons cream of tartar**
½ **cup coconut**
¼ **cup orange juice**
½ **cup mashed banana**
1 **teaspoon vanilla**
½ **cup honey**
1 **tablespoon orange rind**
1 **medium apple, grated**
1 **large or 2 medium eggs or 3 stiffly beaten**
 egg whites

Sift carob powder, flour, bicarb soda and cream of tartar, then add coconut. Blend orange juice, banana, vanilla, honey and rind. Add to flour mixture, stirring well. Stir in grated apple and add beaten eggs or fold in egg whites. Pour mixture into a lightly greased loaf tin and bake 45-50 minutes in a moderate oven.

Christmas Cake

Free of dairy products, wheat, corn, sugar, eggs, soy and nightshades.

250 g sultanas
250 g currants
250 g raisins, chopped
60 g dried apricots, chopped
90 g prunes, chopped
90 g red glace cherries, chopped (wash to
    remove the syrup)
rind and juice 1 orange
rind and juice 1 lemon
¼ cup sherry
1 cup chopped almonds or brazil nuts
1 large grated apple
1 large grated carrot
1 cup ground sunflower seeds
3 cups dry mashed steamed pumpkin
1 cup buckwheat flour
2 cups brown rice flour
2 teaspoons bicarb soda
1 teaspoon nutmeg
1 teaspoon cinnamon
½-¾ cup unsweetened pineapple juice or
    apple juice
blanched almonds for decorating cake if
    desired

Combine sultanas, currants, raisins, apricots, prunes, cherries, orange rind and juice, lemon rind and juice and sherry, and leave to soak as long as desired. After soaking, add chopped nuts, grated apple and carrot and ground sunflower seeds, mixing well with fruit. Add mashed pumpkin, mixing well. Sift flours, bicarb soda, cinnamon and nutmeg and stir into cake. Lastly add fruit juice, mixing all ingredients well together. Lightly grease a large round or square cake tin and line with a layer of brown paper. Spoon mixture into tin. Decorate top with blanched almonds if desired. Bake in a moderate oven for 1 hour, then reduce heat to 150°C and bake 1-1½ hours longer or till cooked.

Buckwheat Cake

Free of dairy products, wheat, yeast, corn, sugar, eggs, soy, orange and nightshades.

1½ cups buckwheat flour
½ teaspoon bicarb soda
1 teaspoon cream of tartar
½ cup ground sunflower seeds
1 cup ground nuts e.g. almonds
½ cup honey
1 cup water
1 green apple, peeled and grated
1 teaspoon cinnamon

Mix together buckwheat flour, bicarb soda, cream of tartar, ground seeds and nuts. Add honey and water, mixing in well. Spoon into a lightly greased round cake tin. Spread grated apple evenly over top of cake and dust with cinnamon. Bake in moderate oven until the centre of cake is firm to touch.

Walnut-Date Loaf

Free of dairy products, wheat, corn, sugar, eggs, orange and nightshades.
Can be made free of yeast if fresh, not dried, dates are used.

1 ¼ **cups water**
¾ **cup chopped dried or fresh dates**
1 **cup chopped walnuts**
1 **teaspoon mixed spice**
1 **tablespoon honey (optional)**
¾ **cup soy flour**
¾ **cup brown rice flour**
1 **teaspoon bicarb soda**
2 **teaspoons cream of tartar**
2 **teaspoons lemon juice**

Bring to boil water, dates, walnuts and mixed spice. Stir in honey and leave to cool. When cool, add flours, bicarb soda, cream of tartar and lemon juice, mixing well. Pour into a lightly greased loaf tin and bake in a moderate oven until firm.

Carrot Cake

Free of dairy products, wheat, yeast, corn, sugar, soy, orange and nightshades.

1 ½ **cups brown rice flour**
1 **teaspoon bicarb soda**
2 **teaspoons cream of tartar**
1 **teaspoon cinnamon**
1 **teaspoon mixed spice**
½ **cup chopped walnuts or pecans**
1 **cup mashed steamed pumpkin**
¼-½ **cup honey**
few drops pure vanilla
1 **cup fine grated carrot**
2 **beaten eggs or 3 stiffly beaten egg**
  whites

Sift first five ingredients. Add nuts. Blend pumpkin, honey and vanilla and add to flour mixture. Stir in grated carrot. Add beaten eggs or fold in egg whites. Pour into a lightly greased cake tin and bake in a moderate oven approximately 1 hour or till cooked.

Before baking spread with grated apple, cinnamon and a drizzle of honey. Alternatively ice with ricotta icing when cool.

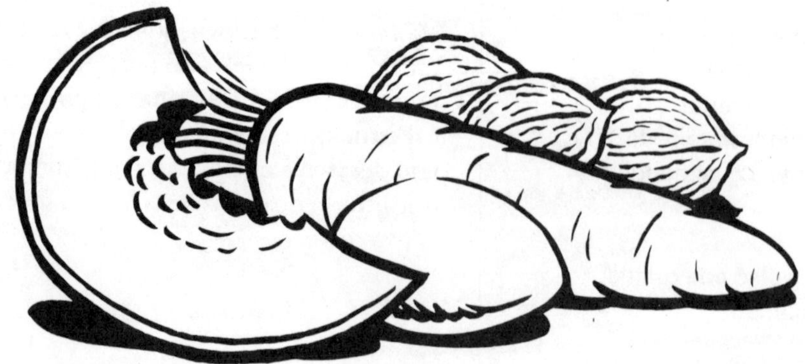

Apple Cake

Free of dairy products, wheat, sugar, eggs, soy, orange and nightshades.

2 cups hot stewed apple (cook apple in
   very little water to which has been
   added a pinch ground cloves)
½ cup honey
1 teaspoon bicarb soda
½ cup chopped nuts
½ cup chopped raisins
1½ tablespoons carob powder
1 cup brown rice flour
½ cup fine cornmeal
½ cup buckwheat flour
½ teaspoon mixed spice
½ teaspoon nutmeg
1 teaspoon cinnamon
1 teaspoon bicarb soda

Add honey and 1 teaspoon bicarb soda to apple (this mixture will become fluffy). Add chopped nuts and raisins to apple mixture. Sift remaining ingredients and stir into apple mixture. Spoon into a lightly greased round cake tin and bake in a moderate oven for 45-50 minutes.

Plain Cake

Free of dairy products, wheat, yeast, corn, sugar, soy, orange and nightshades.

1¾ cups brown rice flour
1 teaspoon bicarb soda
2 teaspoons cream of tartar
1 cup ground almonds
¼-½ cup honey
few drops vanilla
1 cup nut milk
2 eggs or 3 stiffly beaten egg whites

Sift flour, bicarb soda and cream of tartar. Add nuts. Blend honey, vanilla, milk and eggs and add to dry ingredients, mixing well. If using egg whites only, fold in last. Pour into a lightly greased round cake tin and bake in a moderate oven till firm to touch in centre.

Apple Tea Cake

Free of dairy products, wheat, yeast, corn, sugar, soy, orange and nightshades.

1 quantity plain cake mixture
1 small Granny Smith apple, peeled and
   sliced thinly
1 teaspoon cinnamon

Pour cake mixture into a lightly greased round cake tin. Arrange apple slices in a pattern over cake and sprinkle with cinnamon. Bake in a moderate oven till cooked.

Butterfly Cakes

Free of wheat, corn, sugar, soy, orange and nightshades.
Can be free of dairy products if ricotta icing is omitted.

**1 quantity plain cake or sponge cake
mixture**
**1 quantity plain ricotta icing or strawberry
topping or lemon spread**

Spoon cake mixture into patty pan papers and place in patty pans. Bake in a moderate oven. Leave to cool then cut a small circle out of the top of each cake. Fill hollow with ricotta icing or strawberry topping or lemon spread. Cut small circle pieces of cake in half, then position like butterfly wings on top of icing.

Pineapple Upside-down Cake

Free of dairy products, wheat, yeast, corn, sugar, soy, orange and nightshades.

**1 quantity plain cake mixture to which has
been added ½ cup desiccated coconut**
1 ½ cups finely chopped fresh pineapple
2 tablespoons freshly grated coconut

Lightly grease a 20 cm round cake tin. Spread pineapple over bottom of tin. Spread cake mixture evenly over pineapple. Bake in a moderate oven till cake is cooked. Remove from oven and cool slightly. Remove cake from tin and sprinkle fresh or desiccated coconut over the pineapple topping.

Lamingtons

Free of dairy products, wheat, yeast, corn, sugar, soy, orange and nightshades.

**1 quantity plain cake or sponge cake
mixture baked in a square or oblong tin**

Coating

1 cup light carob powder
1 cup water
2-3 tablespoons honey
desiccated coconut

Bake cake and leave to cool. Cut into rectangular shapes about 4.5 cm x 3.5 cm. Bring carob powder and water to the boil and simmer till thickened. Add honey and leave to cool. Holding each cake piece on a fork, spoon coating over and spread with a knife to make a thin layer. Roll in coconut.

Pikelets

Free of dairy products, wheat, corn, sugar, soy, orange and nightshades.
Can be made free of yeast if apple cider vinegar is omitted.

---

1 cup brown rice flour
¼ teaspoon bicarb soda
½ teaspoon cream of tartar
½-¾ cup nut milk
1 teaspoon honey
**1 teaspoon lemon juice or apple cider
vinegar**
1 egg or 2 egg whites, beaten stiffly

Mix dry ingredients together. Beat egg, nut milk, honey and lemon juice together and add to dry ingredients, mixing well. If using egg whites, fold in last. Heat pan and add a little ghee. Drop spoonfuls onto a pan and cook one side till bubbles appear. Turn and briefly cook other side.

Serve with berry jam and ricotta cream or cashew cream.

Sponge Cake

Free of dairy products, wheat, yeast, sugar, soy, orange and nightshades.
Can be free of corn if cornflour not used.

1 cup brown rice flour
½ cup very fine millet flour or cornflour
1 teaspoon bicarb soda
2 teaspoons cream of tartar
⅓ cup honey or maple syrup
¼ cup nut milk
5 eggs, separated

Sift dry ingredients 2 or 3 times. Blend honey, nut milk and egg yolks and stir into flour. Beat egg whites with 1 teaspoon cream of tartar till stiff, then fold into flour and yolk mixture. Pour into 2 small lightly greased round cake tins and bake in a moderate oven till cooked. When cakes are cool, sandwich together using caramel icing as a filling (see Icings section) or lemon or strawberry topping or ricotta icing.

Peanut Butter Cake

Free of dairy products, wheat, yeast, sugar, corn, soy, orange and nightshades.

1 cup brown rice flour
1 teaspoon bicarb soda
2 teaspoons cream of tartar
¼ cup walnut pieces
1 grated apple
½ cup peanut butter
½ cup honey
1 teaspoon vanilla
2 beaten eggs or 3 stiffly beaten egg
    whites

Sift together flour, bicarb soda and cream of tartar. Stir in walnut pieces and grated apple. Beat honey and peanut butter together, then add vanilla and eggs. (If using egg whites only, fold in last.) Combine peanut mixture with flour. Bake in a lightly greased round cake tin in a moderate oven. Leave to cool, then ice with peanut butter icing — see Icings section. Decorate with walnuts.

Variation:

Substitute cashew paste for peanut butter and ice cake with coffee icing.

Festive Icecream Cake

Free of dairy products, wheat, corn, sugar, orange and nightshades.
May be made free of eggs.

This spectacular and delicious cake has to be made over 2 or 3 days. It is built up in 9 layers of Icecream, Berry Topping and Carob Dessert Cake.

Make in a round container 20cm wide and at least 11cm deep.

Icecream

You will need 3 quantities but only make
    one at a time.
2 cups frozen raspberries
½ large avocado or 1 small avocado
1 large banana
1 tablespoon tahini
2 tablespoons honey

Blend ingredients thoroughly and freeze.

Berry Topping

Carob Dessert Cake

This cake can be made without egg whites. Make one quantity of mixture (recipe in Desserts section). Divide and bake in two 20cm cake tins in a moderate oven.

Variation 1:

Make the middle layer Carob Icecream
1 cup dark grape juice
⅓ cup coconut cream
1 small banana
2 tablespoons tahini
2 tablespoons carob powder

Variation 2:

Make a smaller cake of 5 layers (Icecream, Berry Topping, Carob Dessert Cake, Berry topping, Icecream).

Use the topping recipe for Berry Slice (see Slices section) to make one quantity. You will need 4 quantities altogether.

To assemble the cake, freeze these 9 layers in this order:

Icecream. Pour one quantity into the container and freeze.

Berry Topping. Spread on quantity over the frozen, or almost frozen Icecream.

Carob Dessert Cake.

Berry Topping.

Icecream. Pour over Berry Topping and freeze.

Berry Topping.

Carob Dessert Cake.

Berry Topping.

Icecream. Pour over Berry Topping and freeze.

Remove the cake from the freezer ½-1 hour (depending on the weather) before serving. Turn it out of the container and halfway through the defrosting time turn it upside down so that it defrosts evenly. Decorate with strawberries and/or piped cashew cream.

Blend ingredients thoroughly and freeze.

ICINGS

Ricotta Icings

Free of wheat, corn, sugar, eggs, soy, orange and nightshades.

¾ **cup ricotta cheese** **2 teaspoons honey** **few drops pure vanilla**	Blend together thoroughly. **Variations:** Passionfruit — add pulp of 1 passionfruit. Carob (brown) — add 1 tablespoon carob powder. Pink — add 1 teaspoon beetroot juice or for a brighter pink add 1 teaspoon raspberry juice (i.e. juice from frozen raspberries). Green — add 1-2 teaspoons parsley or spinach juice. Yellow — add 2 teaspoons carrot juice.

Peanut Butter Icing

Free of dairy products, wheat, yeast, soy, corn, sugar, eggs, orange and nightshades.

½ **cup very smooth peanut butter** ¼ **cup honey** ¼ **cup carob powder** **1 teaspoon vanilla** **a little hot water to make into a spreadable consistency**	Mix well together till smooth.

Coffee Icing

Free of dairy products, wheat, yeast, soy, corn, eggs, sugar, orange and nightshades.

½ **cup smooth cashew paste** **2 tablespoons honey or maple syrup** **sufficient cereal coffee powder to give a coffee flavour**	Mix ingredients well till smooth.

Caramel Icing

Free of dairy products, wheat, yeast, soy, corn, sugar, eggs, orange and nightshades.

½ **cup smooth cashew paste**
1 **tablespoon honey**
1 **tablespoon maple syrup**
½ **teaspoon pure vanilla**

Mix well together till smooth.

Carob Topping
(See Carob Dessert Cake in Dessert section.)

SLICES AND BISCUITS

These are favourites with children and can be included in the school lunch box, or served for afternoon tea with friends.

Carob Slice

Free of dairy products, wheat, yeast, corn, sugar, eggs, soy, orange and nightshades.

Base

1 cup ground almonds
½ cup chopped almonds
½ cup coconut
2 tablespoons carob powder
1 tablespoon honey
½ cup tahini

Mix ingredients together well, and press into a pie dish, then refrigerate.

Topping

¼ cup honey
¼ cup tahini
½ cup carob powder

Melt honey, then stir in tahini. Add carob, mixing well. Press over base with a knife dipped in hot water. Refrigerate until firm, then cut into small squares.

Sesame Slice

Free of dairy products, wheat, yeast, corn, sugar, eggs, soy, orange and nightshades.

Base

¾ cup rolled millet
¾ cup coconut
¼ cup sesame seeds, ground
3 tablespoons honey
½ cup tahini (or enough to allow mixture to
    hold together)

Combine ingredients. Press into an 18 cm square casserole dish and bake for 15 minutes in a moderate oven. Leave to cool before adding topping.

Topping

2 cups boiling water
1 cup honey
2 tablespoons agar* flakes
½ cup cold water
1 tablespoon lemon juice

Combine water, honey and agar in saucepan and heat until agar is dissolved. Add cold water and lemon juice and leave till cool and beginning to set. Spoon gently over base and refrigerate. Cut into small squares.

Note: This slice should be used sparingly because of its high honey content.
    * See note on agar in glossary.

Berry Slice

Free of dairy products, wheat, yeast, corn, sugar, soy, eggs, orange and nightshades.

Base

2 cups brown rice flour
½ cup honey
¾ cup tahini
2-3 drops pure almond essence

Mix ingredients together and press into a tray.

Topping

1 cup strawberries
1 cup blackberries
1-3 tablespoons honey
1 ½ tablespoons arrowroot mixed in
    2 tablespoons water

Heat berries and honey. When boiling, lower heat and stir in arrowroot until mixture is thick, then remove from heat. When cool spread over base. Decorate with almonds and coconut. Bake in a moderate oven for approximately 15 minutes or until almonds are lightly browned.

Muesli Slice

Free of dairy products, wheat, corn, sugar, eggs, soy, orange and nightshades.

½ cup rolled millet
2 cups rolled oats or puffed millet
1 cup sunflower seeds
½ cup brown rice flour
¼ cup currants or chopped fresh dates
¼ cup finely chopped dried apricots
2 cups almonds
⅓ cup honey
⅓ cup hot water

Mix together rolled millet, rolled oats or puffed millet, sunflower seeds, brown rice flour, currants and apricots. Grind almonds to a paste. Add almond paste, honey and hot water to dry mixture, mixing all ingredients well together. Spread onto a lightly greased tray. Bake in a moderate oven until lightly browned. Cool, then refrigerate before slicing.

Tahini Cookies

Free of dairy products, wheat, yeast, corn, sugar, soy, orange and nightshades.

6 tablespoons tahini
⅓ cup honey
1 egg
1 cup rice flakes
½ cup coconut
½ cup sunflower seeds

Mix together tahini and honey. Add remaining ingredients, stirring well. Drop tablespoonfuls onto a well greased tray and bake till brown but not overcooked.

Almond Loaf

Free of dairy products, wheat, yeast, corn, sugar, soy, orange and nightshades.

3 egg whites
pinch cream of tartar
¼-½ cup honey
few drops almond essence
1 cup brown rice flour (sifted if desired)
½ cup blanched almonds, halved

Beat egg whites with cream of tartar. Gradually beat in honey and almond essence until the mixture is of meringue consistency, forming thick peaks. Fold in sifted flour and almonds. Spoon into a lightly greased loaf tin and bake in a moderate oven 30-40 minutes. Leave in the tin until completely cold or set aside 1-2 days. Using a sharp knife, slice the bread thinly. Place on a tray and bake in a moderately slow oven until lightly browned.

Gingerbread Men or Cookies

Free of dairy products, wheat, yeast, corn, sugar, eggs, soy and nightshades. *24 cookies or 5 men*

½ **cup brown rice flour**
½ **cup barley flour**
¼ **teaspoon bicarb soda**
½ **teaspoon cream of tartar**
½-1 **teaspoon ground ginger or**
   2 teaspoons carob powder
½ **cup pecans ground till oily**
1 **tablespoon honey**
1 **tablespoon maple syrup**
2 **tablespoons orange juice**
2 **teaspoons grated orange rind**

Sift dry ingredients. Rub in the ground nuts. Add honey, maple syrup, orange juice and orange rind. Knead lightly and divide into halves. Roll out thinly on a floured board. Cut into shapes. Place on a lightly greased tray and bake 15-20 minutes in a moderate oven.

Makes about 2 dozen thinly rolled cookies or 5 x 13 cm thick men.

Anzac Biscuits

Free of dairy products, wheat, yeast, corn, sugar, eggs, soy, orange and nightshades.

1 **cup rolled oats**
¼ **cup coconut**
½ **cup brown rice flour**
½ **cup barley flour**
1 **cup pecans or almonds, ground**
2-3 **tablespoons honey**
¼-⅓ **cup hot water**

Combine oats, coconut, brown rice flour and barley flour in a bowl. Rub in the nuts and then add the honey and water. Roll into balls, then flatten between hands and place on a lightly greased tray. Bake in a moderate oven till lightly browned.

Savoury Crackers

Free of dairy products, wheat, corn, sugar, eggs, orange and nightshades.

1 **cup brown rice flour**
½ **cup ground almonds**
1 **tablespoon finely chopped onion**
2 **teaspoons tamari**
½ **teaspoon onion powder**
½ **cup water**
sesame seeds or poppy seeds

Mix together flour, almonds, onion, tamari and onion powder. Add water, mixing all ingredients well together to form a dough. Refrigerate till chilled to make dough easier to handle. Roll dough out thinly on a well-floured board or bench. Press sesame seeds or poppy seeds into the dough using fingers. Cut dough into strips 1 ½ cm wide, then cut each strip diagonally several times to make diamond shapes or cut with cookie cutters. Place on a lightly greased or floured tray and bake in a moderate oven until biscuits are crisp and lightly browned.

Serve as pre-dinner nibbles or as a snack for children's playlunches.

Macaroons

Free of dairy products, wheat, yeast, corn, sugar, soy, orange and nightshades.

4 egg whites
½-1 cup honey or maple syrup
2 teaspoons vanilla
few drops almond essence
1 tablespoon brown rice flour
1 cup ground almonds
2 cups coconut

Beat egg whites until stiff. Slowly add maple syrup or honey. Mix in remaining ingredients. Drop by spoonfuls onto a well greased tray. Bake in a slow oven for ½ hour and remove from tray when cool.

Note: If not crisp when cold, return to oven and cook approximately 15 minutes more.

Gluten Free Biscuits

Free of dairy products, wheat, yeast, corn, sugar, eggs, soy, orange and nightshades.

1 cup puffed millet
¼ cup coconut
1 cup brown rice flour
½ teaspoon cream of tartar
1 cup pecans or cashews, ground
3 tablespoons honey
3 tablespoons boiling water
½ teaspoon bicarb soda

Combine millet, coconut, flour and cream of tartar. Rub in the nuts. Melt honey in the water and add bicarb soda. Add to dry ingredients, mixing well. Roll into small balls and place on a lightly greased tray. Flatten with a fork. Bake in a moderate oven till lightly browned.

Carob Brownies

Free of dairy products, wheat, corn, sugar, soy, orange and nightshades.

¼ cup carob powder
1 cup brown rice flour or barley flour
1 teaspoon bicarb soda
2 teaspoons cream of tartar
½ cup chopped raisins
½ cup chopped nuts
1 grated apple
¼-½ cup honey or maple syrup
**2 beaten eggs or 2 stiffly beaten egg
    whites**

Sift first four ingredients. Add raisins, nuts and apple. Mix together or blend honey and eggs and add to flour mixture. (If using egg whites only, fold in last.) Bake in a lightly greased tray in a moderate oven till cooked. Cool, then ice with coffee icing or caramel icing (see Icing section), or ice with carob topping (see Dessert section). Cut into squares and decorate with walnuts or pecans.

Sesame Squares

Free of dairy products, wheat, soy, corn, sugar, orange, eggs and nightshades.
Can be free of yeast by omitting raisins.

200 g sesame seeds
1 cup coconut
⅓ cup peanut butter
½ cup honey
½ teaspoon vanilla
½ cup chopped nuts
1 cup rolled oats
½ cup raisins, chopped (optional)

Mix all ingredients together thoroughly. Press into greased square cake tin. Bake in moderate oven until lightly browned, approx. 30 minutes. When cold cut into squares.

Butterfly Cakes (p108) filled with Ricotta Cream (p111)
Carob Men (p116) Almond Loaf (p115) Strawberry Tarts (p83)
and Lemon Tarts (p82) with Ricotta Cream

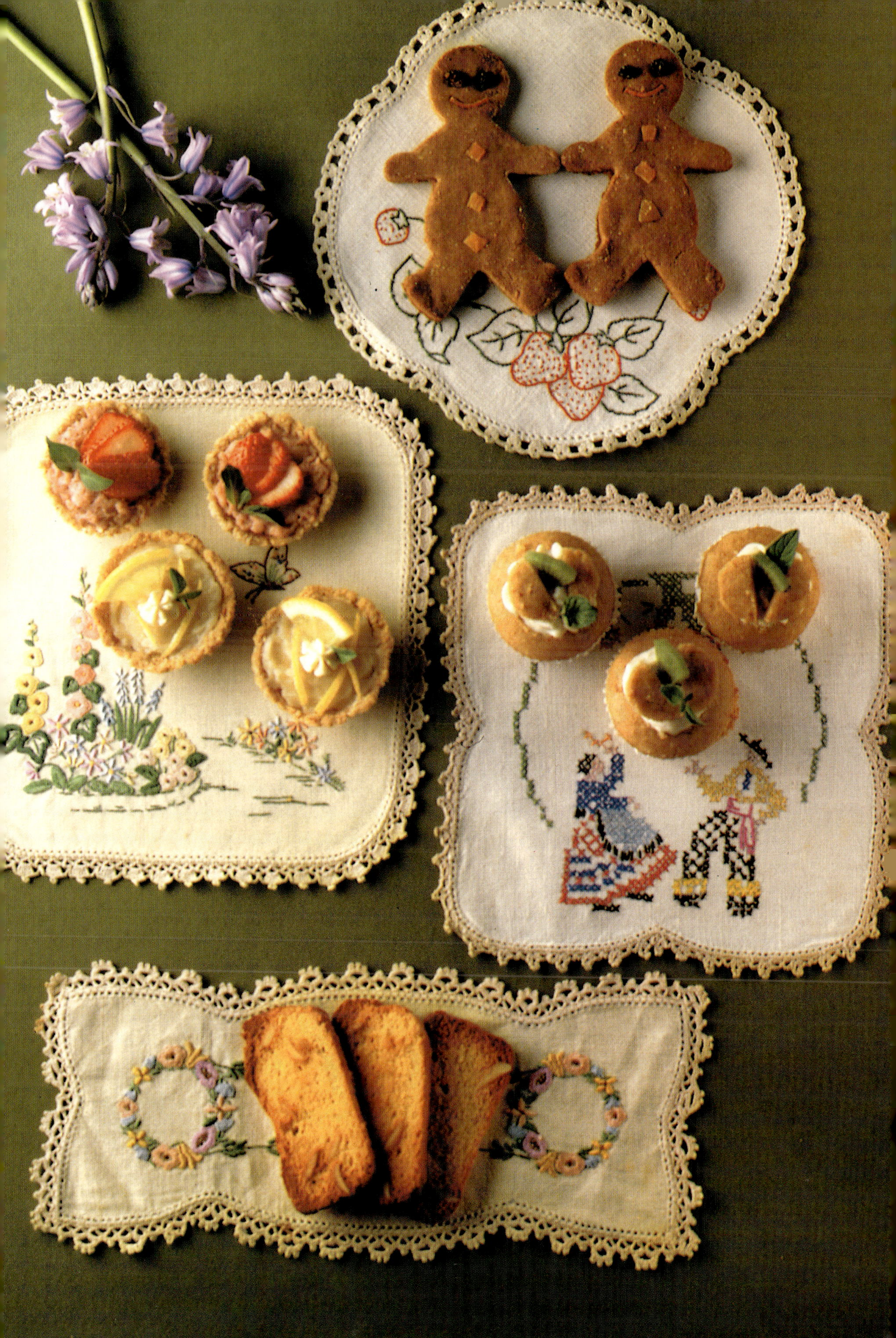

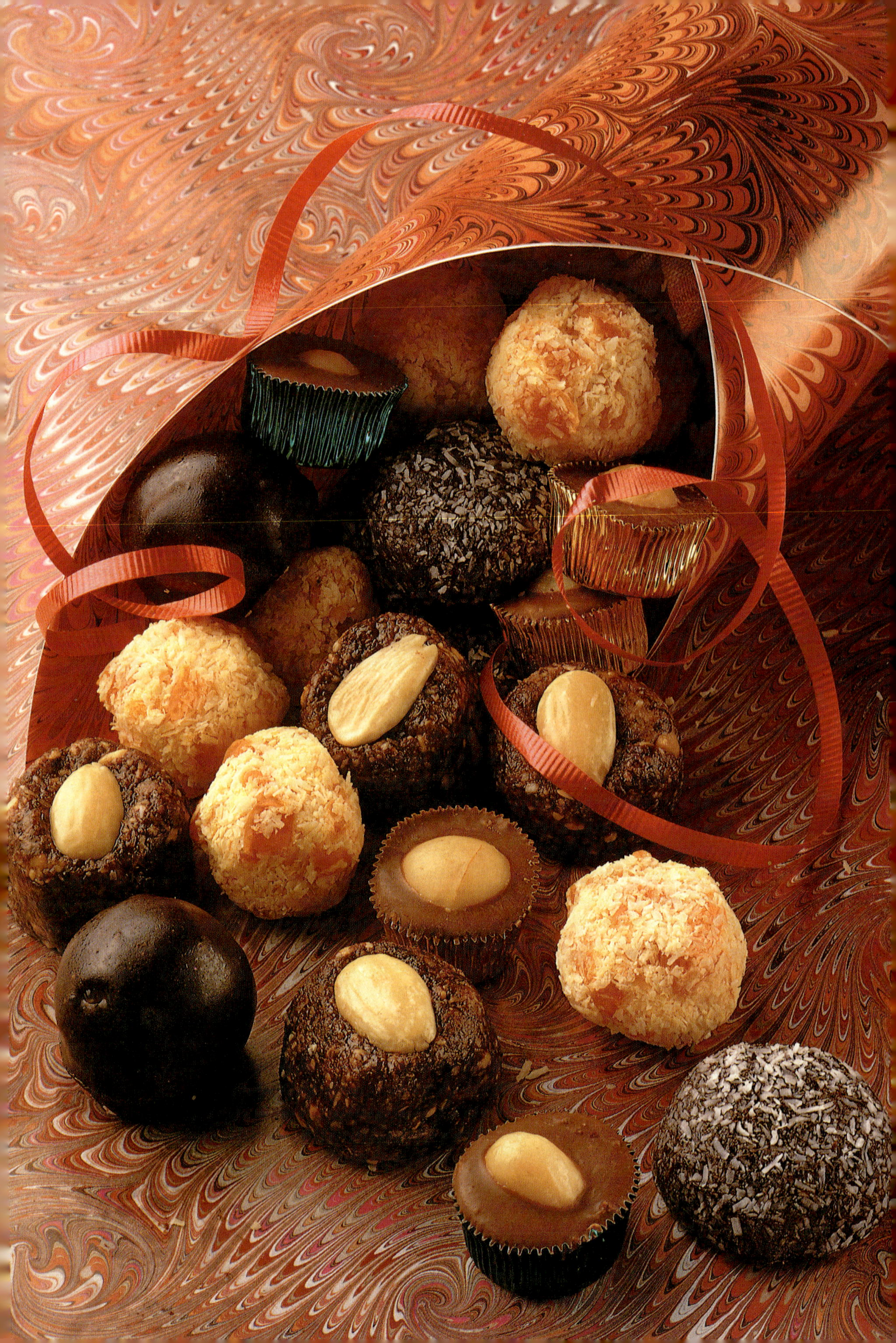

CONFECTIONERY

These sweets are popular with children and adults alike and are suitable for parties, entertaining and gifts.

Carob Peppermint Balls

Free of dairy products, wheat, yeast, corn, sugar, eggs, soy, orange and nightshades.

¼ **cup honey** ¼ **cup tahini** ½ **cup carob powder** **few drops peppermint oil**	Melt honey over low heat. Stir in tahini, then carob powder and peppermint, mixing well together. Roll into small balls, then roll in coconut and refrigerate.

Halva

Free of dairy products, wheat, yeast, corn, sugar, eggs, soy, orange and nightshades.

1 ½ cups hulled sesame seeds **1 tablespoon honey**	Grind seeds into a fine meal. Work in honey. Roll into small balls, then roll in sesame seeds or coconut.

Fruit and Nut Balls

Free of dairy products, wheat, corn, sugar, eggs, soy, orange and nightshades.

½ **cup finely chopped dried figs or prunes** ½ **cup finely chopped dates** ½ **cup finely chopped dried apricots** **1 tablespoon honey** ½ **cup finely chopped pecans** ½ **cup ground almonds**	Mix ingredients thoroughly together. Roll into small balls.

Carob Fudge Balls, Carob Peppermint Balls, Apricot Coconut Balls, Carob
Coated Nut Balls (pp119-120) Macadamias in Carob Cases (p142)

Apricot-Coconut Balls

Free of dairy products, wheat, corn, sugar, eggs, soy and nightshades.

¾ cup dried apricots soaked in boiling
water till soft
½ teaspoon lemon juice
1 tablespoon orange juice
¾ cup coconut
1 teaspoon orange rind

Drain water from apricots and chop finely. Mix with remaining ingredients. Roll into small balls, then roll in coconut.

Carob Fudge Balls

Free of dairy products, wheat, yeast, corn, sugar, eggs, soy, orange and nightshades.

½ cup nut butter e.g. almond or cashew or
hazelnut
¼ cup honey
¼ cup carob powder
1 teaspoon vanilla
1 cup coconut

Mix all ingredients together and roll into small balls. Refrigerate.

Carob Coated Nut Balls

Free of dairy products, wheat, corn, sugar, eggs, soy and nightshades. Can be free of yeast if apricots are omitted and fresh dates are used.

Nut Balls

1 cup ground almonds
1 cup ground hazelnuts
1 cup ground pecans
¾ cup finely chopped dried apricots (soak
   in orange juice first to soften) or
   chopped fresh dates
1 teaspoon pure orange essence or
   2 teaspoons cointreau
1 teaspoon orange rind
1 teaspoon maple syrup

Mix ingredients together well and shape into balls.

Carob Coating

⅓ cup carob powder
2 tablespoons orange juice
¼ cup honey
1 heaped tablespoon agar* flakes
½ cup water

Mix together carob powder, orange juice and honey. Place agar flakes and water in saucepan, bring to boil and simmer till flakes are dissolved. Stir agar and water mixture into carob mixture and let cool slightly. Quickly dip nut balls into carob mixture, coating evenly, and place on a plate to set.

   * See note on agar in glossary.

FROZEN TREATS

Popsicles

These are not only a treat for children, but a positive addition to a nutritious diet.

Banana

Free of dairy products, wheat, yeast, corn, sugar, eggs, soy, orange and nightshades.

Halve large bananas or use 1 Lady Finger. Insert a paddlepop (obtainable from newsagents or craft shops). Wrap in plastic and freeze.

Carob Frozen Banana

Free of wheat, yeast, corn, sugar, eggs, soy (unless carob block contains lecithin), orange and nightshades.

A special treat. Prepare bananas as above. Melt a block of unsweetened carob and dip in tip of bananas. Freeze.

Nutty Frozen Banana

Free of dairy products, wheat, yeast, corn, sugar, eggs, soy, orange and nightshades.

Prepare bananas as above. Dip in honey or maple syrup and roll in finely chopped pecan nuts. Freeze.

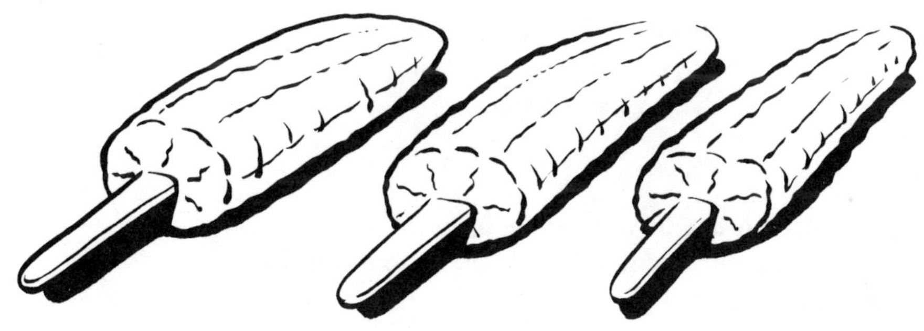

Fruity Icypoles

A great variety of icypoles can be made from fruit purees and juices
either singly or in combination. A few suggestions are listed below.
Yoghurt or nut butters may be added for a creamier taste. Fruit juices —
apple, pear, pineapple, watermelon and grape all make excellent
icypoles.

Strawberry

Puree 1 punnet of strawberries or other berries and mix with 1 cup water
or fruit juice, e.g. orange, apple, pear. Freeze in moulds.

Mango

Puree with a little orange juice. Add 1-2 tablespoons of coconut cream
or yoghurt per 1 cup puree to give a creamy texture.

Pineapple

Mash ripe pineapple and combine with passionfruit. Freeze.

Banana

Mash banana with apple juice and add passionfruit. Freeze.

Tropical freeze

See Desserts section. Pour into moulds and freeze.

Frozen Whole Fruits

Grapes

Grapes freeze well and keep for weeks. They can be defrosted, but served
frozen they make wonderful hot-weather treats for children and adults
alike. The larger varieties are the most successful.

Navel oranges

Sweet oranges in peak condition are a great favourite with children on
hot days. Freeze orange, whole and unpeeled. Allow to soften slightly
and cut into halves or quarters.

Fruit Juice Sherbets

Children love this simple treat. Freeze a quantity of pineapple or apple
juice. Allow to soften slightly and blend into a sherbet in the processor.
Place in a cup and serve with a spoon.

Frozen Carob Moulds
Free of dairy products, wheat, yeast, corn, sugar, eggs, soy, orange and nightshades.

2 teaspoons agar* flakes
½ cup apple juice
1 tablespoon honey or maple syrup
2 teaspoons arrowroot
¼ cup soymilk, or thick nut milk
¼ cup tahini
1 teaspoon vanilla
½ cup soymilk, or thick nut milk
½ cup carob powder

Combine agar, juice and honey in a pan. Bring to the
boil, then simmer gently until agar has dissolved. Mix
arrowroot in ¼ cup milk and add to agar mixture,
stirring over a low heat until thickened. Combine
tahini, vanilla and ½ cup milk together and stir into
agar mixture. Add carob and mix well — sift if there
are lumps. Pour into small moulds, e.g. chocolate
moulds or icypole containers and freeze. When
frozen, carefully run a knife around inside edge of
moulds and gently lift the mixture out.

Serve immediately, as they will melt fairly quickly.

* See note on agar in glossary.

BEVERAGES

Beverages are not only an essential part of maintaining health but are also a focal point of social gatherings. They are thus an important part of our diet and our way of life. Below are some suggestions for nutritious and delicious juices, teas and shakes.

JUICES

Freshly juiced fruits and vegetables can be drunk pure or diluted 50 per cent with water or mineral water and served with tinkling ice cubes if desired.

Fruit Juices

Apple

Probably made best from Granny Smiths which have a firmer texture than many apples. Some sprigs of mint or slices of mango can be put through with the apple to give delightfully different flavours.

Mandarins

A good alternative to oranges when in season. Peel and juice as other fruits.

Pineapple, watermelon, strawberry and grape

These are all delicious spring and summer juices. White or black grapes are equally suitable; pineapple juice with coconut milk is a beautiful combination and watermelon will delight with fresh colour and flavour.

Vegetable juices

Vegetable juices can be mixed to give interesting and health promoting combinations. Carrots make an excellent base for them. Rich in Vitamin A, carrot juice is an excellent tonic and cleanser; drink alone or with celery, spinach, parsley or beetroot. Green juice can be made from any mixtures of green vegetables. Wheatgrass juice can be added if desired.

HERB TEA AND COFFEE SUBSTITUTES

There are many substitutes for the more usual tea and coffee. A visit to any health food store or even some supermarkets will yield a wide choice. Coffee — cereal based or dandelion root coffee substitutes are available. They have a coffee-like flavour, in many cases, and are all caffeine free. Dandelion root can be percolated like coffee and is not only delicious but is known as an excellent liver cleanser.

Tea

A wide range of herb teas are available and can be prepared from dried herbs e.g. bulk or tea bags, or as infusions fresh from the garden. To make an infusion, take several sprigs of the desired herb, e.g. peppermint, rosemary, lemon grass. Pour over boiling water and allow to stand at least 5 minutes for flavour to develop.

All herb teas are refreshing and have individual health-giving properties. Your choice will depend on taste or medical advice. All can be served warm to hot but some such as lemon grass and peppermint are refreshing as an iced summer drink. Simply steep in boiling water, allow to stand for 5-15 minutes, then refrigerate.

MILK DRINKS

Dairy products are a problem for many people. Goat's milk makes an
excellent alternative to cow's milk but some people are either intolerant
of it or wish to keep their diet milk free. Other milks can be prepared
from nuts and seeds and soybeans. They are both nutritious and delicious
used as a basis for drinks, over mueslis or cereals or in baking.

Basic Nut/Seed Milk

Free of dairy products, wheat, yeast, corn, sugar, eggs, soy, orange and nightshades.

2 cups pure water **¼-½ cup almonds or other nuts or sesame or sunflower seeds** **1 teaspoon honey (optional)**	Blend for 1-2 minutes and strain. A thicker nut milk can be made by blending 1 cup of nuts with 1 cup water.

Soya Milk

Free of dairy products, wheat, yeast, corn, sugar, eggs, orange and nightshades.

1 cup soya flour **1 litre water** **1 vanilla bean (optional)**	By far the easiest way is to buy powdered lactose-free soy milk ready for use but below is a recipe should you wish to prepare your own. Mix the flour to a paste with a little of the water and then add the rest. Place in a pan with the vanilla bean and heat to just below boiling point, stirring constantly. Do not allow to boil. Simmer for 15 minutes and strain. Any of the above milks can be used to make tasty drinks and shakes which will be greatly appreciated by children with dairy allergies.

Banana or Strawberry Milkshake

Free of dairy products, wheat, yeast, corn, sugar, eggs, soy, orange and nightshades.

2 cups milk substitute **1 medium banana or ½ cup strawberries** **½-1 teaspoon vanilla** **1 teaspoon to 1 tablespoon honey or maple syrup** **ice cubes**	Blend at high speed, then sprinkle with cinnamon or use ¼ teaspoon in the shake.

Carob Drink or Milkshake

Free of dairy products, wheat, yeast, corn, sugar, eggs, soy, orange and nightshades.

1 cup milk substitute
2 teaspoons carob powder
1 teaspoon to 1 tablespoon honey
½ teaspoon vanilla or ¼ teaspoon nutmeg
  or cinnamon

A favourite with children. In hot weather blend with icecubes or make as a hot drink in winter or before bedtime.

Blend lightly and heat if desired.

Coconut Milk

Coconut milk can be bought unsweetened or made by pouring 1 cup boiling water over 1 cup freshly grated coconut or 1 cup boiling water over ½-1 cup desiccated coconut. Leave to stand 1 hour, then squeeze milk out using a cheesecloth or press through a strainer. The milk can be used in baking or poured over mueslis or mixed with pineapple juice.

Tropical Fruit Punch

Free of dairy products, wheat, yeast, corn, sugar, eggs, soy, orange and nightshades.

1 large pineapple, skin removed and
  chopped, or 2 cups pineapple juice
3 litres tropical fruit juice (unsweetened),
  or juice your own using apples,
  mangoes, pineapple etc.
a little ground ginger to taste (optional)
chopped fresh mint leaves to garnish
pulp 10 passionfruit
1 litre soda water

Puree pineapple in blender then mix with juice, ginger, mint and passionfruit. Add soda water just before serving.
  Serve chilled with or without crushed ice.

Lemonade

Free of dairy products, wheat, yeast, corn, sugar, eggs, soy, orange and nightshades.

2 cups lemon grass tea
2-3 tablespoons lemon juice
1 tablespoon honey
½ cup soda water
ice blocks

Mix together tea, lemon juice and honey. Just before serving add soda water and ice cubes.

Potassium Broth

Free of dairy products, wheat, yeast, corn, sugar, eggs, soy and orange.
Can be free of nightshades if sweet potatoes are used instead of white potatoes.

Finely chop 2 potatoes or sweet potatoes as a base for the broth. Add
other finely chopped vegetables, e.g. carrots, celery and celery leaves,
parsley, swede, parsnip, beetroot and spinach. Avoid onions and
cabbage. Place vegetables in a pan with water to cover and simmer for
half an hour. Leave to stand a further 30 minutes, then strain and drink.
It can be refrigerated and used over 1-2 days.

ENTERTAINING

Once you have moved onto an allergy-planned health-promoting diet, entertaining can cause some concern. What do you serve Aunty whose great love at afternoon tea time is fluffy sponge cake with jam and cream filling; or the new boss you wish to impress but who you know loves a meal of oysters, filet mignon with red wine and profiteroles.

You can, if you wish, prepare a range of foods which encompass both your style of eating and your guests', but that means you are going to have to go out and buy ingredients such as white flour and sugar, which you have progressively eliminated from your pantry and which you probably won't use for some time. It also can make for a rather odd meal and a lot of extra work when you would wish to be as relaxed as possible and enjoy your guests.

Below are some suggestions for such occasions which we feel will help solve the problem for you as they have for us. Remember that increasingly people are becoming aware of healthier styles of eating and are often interested in them.

Setting

One of the most important aspects of eating in company is the setting. A pleasant environment, an attractive table setting and deliciously prepared natural fresh foods are the best possible ingredients for a pleasant get-together. An attractive dining room, a cheerful sunny kitchen, a shaded table in the garden or even a rug under a tree on the lawn are all fine places for a meal. Any meal can be an occasion for entertaining, even breakfast. One of the great pleasures of eating is sharing a meal in congenial company with good conversation and laughter whether it is a formal meal at a candlelit dining table, an impromptu get-together with friends or a picnic in the garden with the children.

Suggestions

Breakfast

Juice
Fresh fruit e.g. Pawpaw boats, Sunshine Breakfast, banana smoothie.
Waffles or muffins with strawberry sauce and maple syrup or lemon spread.
Dandelion coffee or herb tea.

Lunch (1)

Baked beans with seed bread and mixed salad.
Fresh fruit platter.

Lunch (2)

Quiche with green salad.
Strawberry jelly with cashew cream or custard apple sauce.

Lunch (3)

Lentil pâté with mixed salad and Ryvita or rice crackers.
Custard apples.

Lunch (4)

Chicken and rice salad served in lettuce leaves.
Sprout salad and coleslaw.
Berry icecream.

Lunch (5)

Avocado soup, chick pea soup or lentil soup; nori sea vegetable.
Chicken spread or curried tofu spread on waffles.

Smorgasbord

Choose from any of the following

Savoury Dishes
Nut terrine
Lentil pâté
Fish and chicken pieces with sweet and sour sauce
Stuffed chicken fillets
Curried eggs
Raw nut mould
Fish and pineapple tartlets
Avocado dip with crackers
Pizza
Fried rice

Salads
Carrot and raisin salad
Green salad
Sprout salad
Purple salad

Breads and crackers
Seed bread
Pumpkin rice bread
Sesame rice waffles
Rye or rice crackers

Desserts
Mango-yoghurt pie
Lemon curd tart
Strawberry jelly
Fruit jelly
Festive icecream cake
Orange slice
Apple pie with cashew cream

Dinners

Choose from any of the following

Hors d'oeuvres
Crudites with dips
Nori rolls
Nibble mix
Rum prunes

Dinner (1)

Entree
Avocado vinaigrette

Main course
Fish fillets with curry sauce and mango, baked potato, steamed broccoli
and carrots julienne.

Dessert
Tropical freeze garnished with mint leaves.

Dinner (2)

Entree
Stuffed mushrooms

Main course
Tofu casserole with rice and green salad.

Dinner (3)

Entree
Pâté with crackers or seed bread.

Main course
Chicken with grapes and macadamia nuts, rice, spinach, carrots.

Dessert
Layered fruit salad with cashew cream, ricotta cream or tahini cream.

BARBECUES

Barbecues are, without doubt, a national institution. They are an excellent means of entertaining small or large groups or for a summer weekend lunch, or dinner for the family. Despite the most commonly served steak, chops and sausages, barbecues do not have to centre on meat.

Some delicious and attractive alternatives are included here, and with the great range of seafood in our fish markets at present we're sure you will find others for yourself.

Barbecued Whole Fish

Free of wheat, corn, sugar, eggs, orange and nightshades.

Basting liquid	
1 tablespoon ghee, melted	Brush fish with sauce and cook on barbecue rack,
1 tablespoon tamari	basting often. Turn once only. Sprinkle with toasted
¼ cup mirin	sesame seeds when nearly done.
2 cloves crushed garlic	Serve with salads, baked potato, and vegetable or
1 tablespoon lemon juice	fruit kebabs.
4 whole small schnapper or bream	

Marinated Calamari Rings

Free of dairy products, wheat, corn, sugar, eggs, orange and nightshades.

Calamari is available just about anywhere today and with a little care in preparation, makes an excellent barbecue either as an entree or main dish. The small squid are considered the most tender, but with preparation the larger sizes can be equally tasty and sometimes are preferable.

Calamari rings	
Marinade	
(make up as much as required)	
1-2 tablespoons tamari	Clean calamari thoroughly, then slice into rings.
1 clove crushed garlic	Marinate for at least 2 hours in the refrigerator.
1 teaspoon grated ginger	Drain. Reserve marinade and thicken into a sauce if
2 tablespoons dry sherry or mirin	desired. Place rings on a lightly greased griddle and
1 tablespoon honey	cook for 10 minutes.

Tofu Kebabs

Free of dairy products, wheat, corn, sugar, eggs and orange.

Approximately 150 g firm tofu per person
green and/or red capsicum
small mushrooms
onions cut in quarters
cherry tomatoes
sufficient quantity of marinade (see
    previous recipe)
bamboo skewers soaked in water for
  30 minutes
a serving of Spicy Nut Sauce (see Sauces
    section)

Marinate tofu in the refrigerator for 2-3 hours. Thread tofu and vegetables onto skewers. Barbecue for 5-10 minutes on a hot griddle or low fire.

Serve with salads, rice and spicy nut sauce.

Golden Nugget Hot Pots

Free of dairy products, wheat, corn, sugar, eggs and orange.

---

3 Golden Nugget pumpkins

Slice off top of pumpkins and scoop out seeds. Chop a variety of vegetables, e.g. onion (1 small-medium), mushrooms (in halves), celery (sliced), tomatoes (1-2, chopped), 1 clove crushed garlic, ¼ cup peas, ½ cup cooked brown rice, 100 g crumbled tofu, cottage cheese or cooked lentils can be added, 1-2 teaspoons chopped fresh oregano, 1-2 teaspoons chopped fresh basil, 2 teaspoons tomato paste, 1 teaspoon tamari.

Briefly saute vegetables in a pan. Add tofu, herbs, rice, tomato paste and tamari. Place inside pumpkin. Add lid and cook on a barbecue (covered variety) or in the oven for approximately 1 hour.

BREAKFASTS

Breakfast can be a simple meal of any fresh seasonal fruit, nuts and seeds or yoghurt. It can be more substantial — the choice will depend on personal preference, seasonal and energy requirements.
In this section we offer you foods from fruits and porridge, to waffles, pancakes and muffins. A range from which the whole family can choose.

MUESLIS

Brown Rice Muesli

Free of dairy products, wheat, corn, sugar, eggs, soy, orange and nightshades.
Free of yeast if raisins or sultanas are omitted.

Serves 1

½ cup cooked brown rice
1 apple peeled and grated or 1 chopped banana
1 tablespoon sunflower seeds
1-2 tablespoons ground or chopped nuts
few raisins or sultanas (optional)

Mix together and serve with nut or soy milk.

Soaked Muesli

Free of dairy products, wheat, yeast, corn, sugar, eggs, orange and nightshades.

Serves 1

½ cup rolled oats or ¼ cup rolled rice
water
¼ cup ground nuts and/or seeds e.g.
unhulled sesame, sunflower or linseed
1 piece fresh fruit

Soak oats or rolled rice overnight in water. Next day add nuts and/or seeds, mixing well. Chop piece of fresh fruit in season and add to muesli.
Serve with nut milk or soy milk if desired.

Variation

Substitute lemon juice and honey for the nut milk.

Festive Icecream Cake (p109)

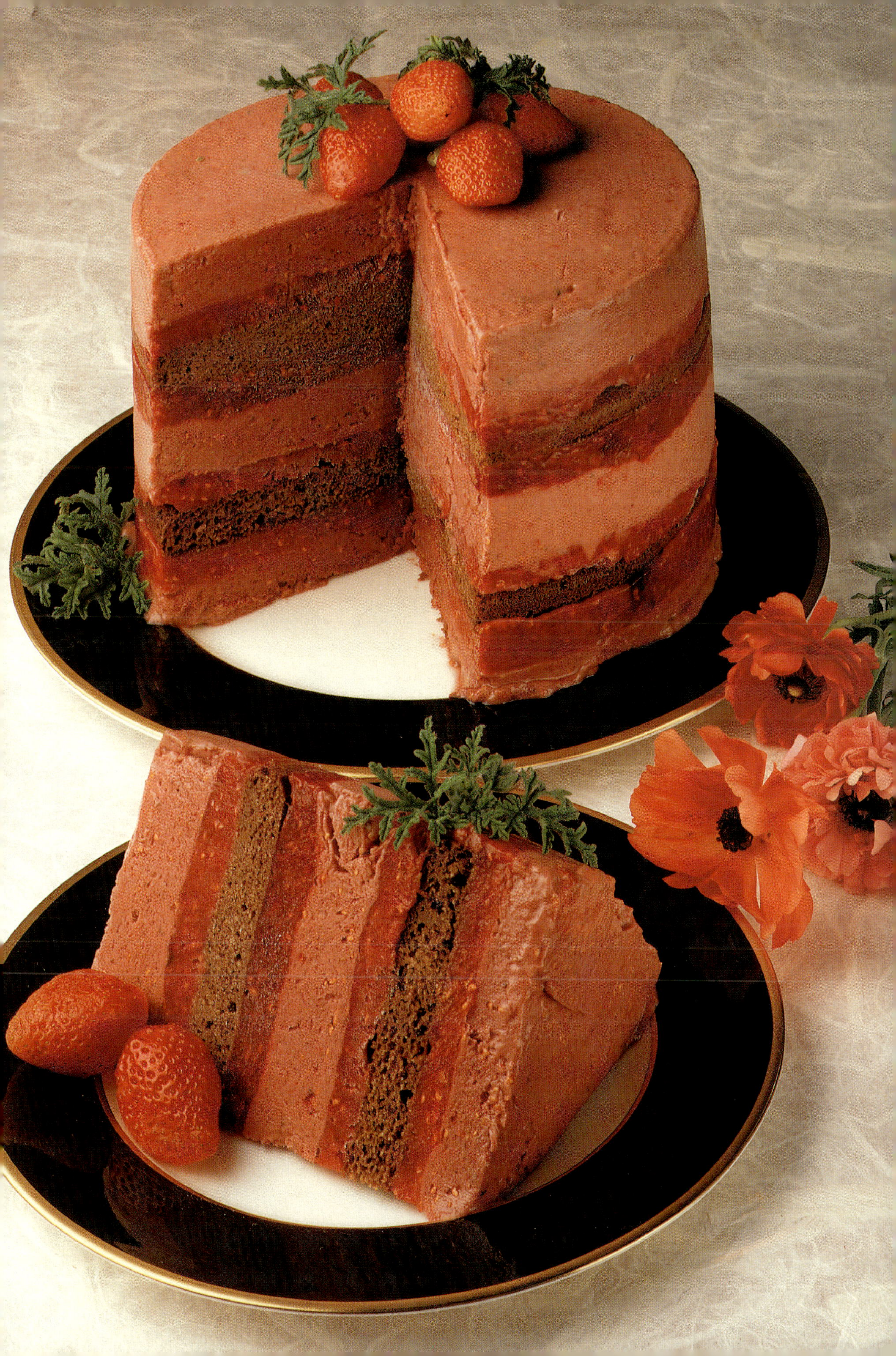

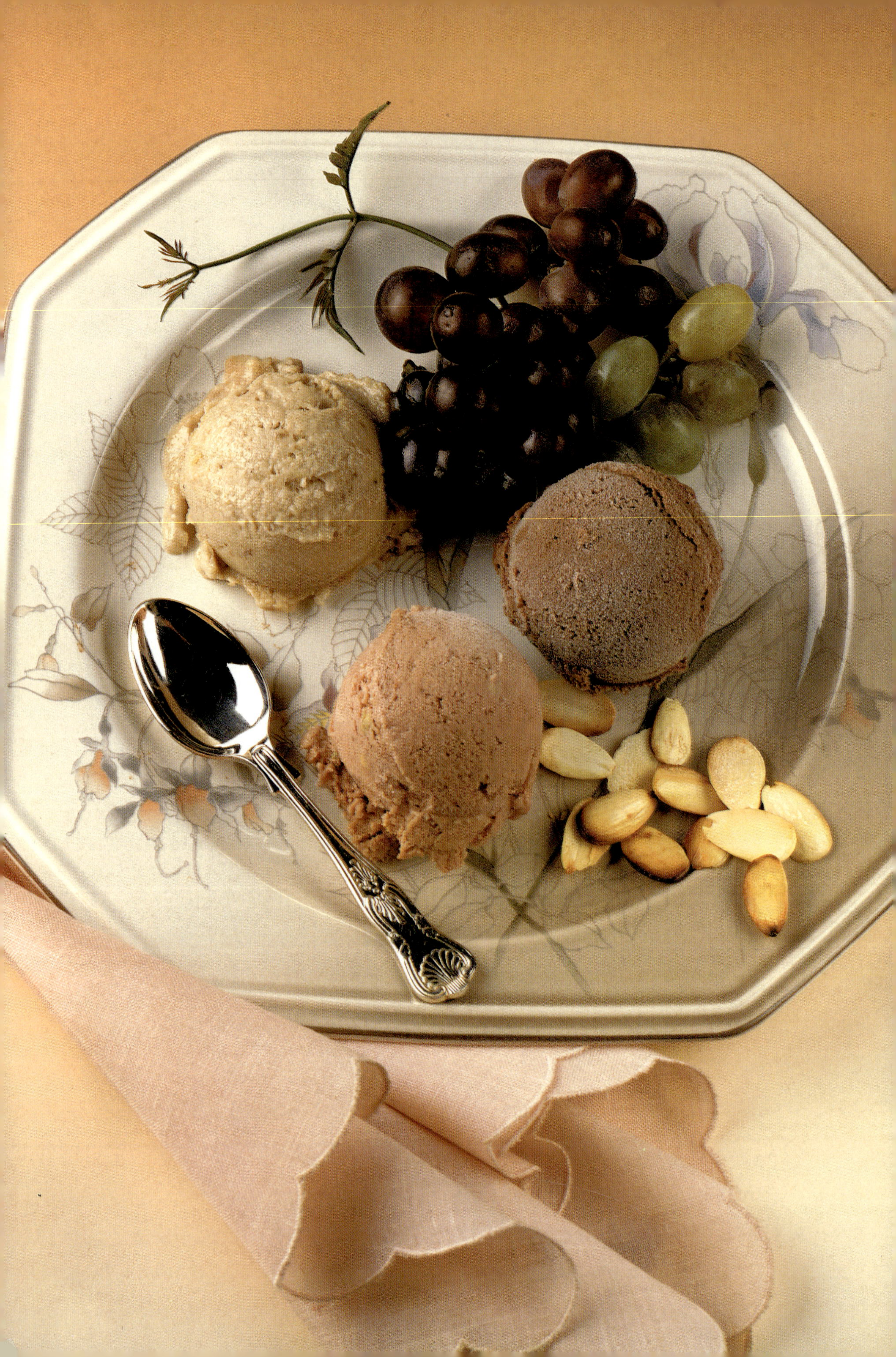

Carob Muesli

Free of dairy products, wheat, corn, sugar, eggs, soy, orange and nightshades.   *Serves 1*

¼ cup puffed millet
2 tablespoons ground almonds
1-2 tablespoons each ground sesame,
pumpkin and sunflower seeds
1 tablespoon sultanas
2 teaspoons carob powder
2 tablespoons coconut

Mix ingredients together and serve with nut or soy milk.

PORRIDGES

Millet Porridge

Free of dairy products, wheat, yeast, corn, sugar, eggs, soy, orange and nightshades.   *Serves 4*

1 cup hulled millet
3 cups hot water

Place millet and water in saucepan, bring to boil then simmer for 10 minutes. Turn off heat and leave until millet has absorbed all the water and become fluffy and soft.

Serve with stewed fruit or chopped bananas, or a few raisins and milk substitute of choice.

Millet Pudding

Free of dairy products, wheat, corn, sugar, eggs, soy, orange and nightshades
Free of yeast if fresh dates are used.   *Serves 4-6*

1 cup whole hulled millet
3 cups nut or soy milk
1 tablespoon honey
½ cup coconut milk
½ cup chopped nuts
½ cup currants (or chopped fresh dates)
¼ cup coconut

Cook millet in nut or soy milk until it boils. Simmer 10-15 mins, then turn off heat and allow to stand until millet has absorbed all the liquid (approximately 10-15 mins). Stir in remaining ingredients. Can be served either hot or cold depending on the season.

Variation:

Stir through Berry Topping (see Slices section).

Icecreams–Strawberry, vanilla and carob flavoured (p75)

Buckwheat Porridge

Free of dairy products, wheat, yeast, corn, sugar, egg, soy, orange and nightshades. *Serves 3-4*

1 cup raw buckwheat groats
2 cups hot water

Place buckwheat and water in saucepan, bring to boil then simmer until buckwheat is soft and the water absorbed. Add more water if necessary.

Serve with substitute milk of choice and any stewed fruit.

Rice Porridge

Free of dairy products, wheat, yeast, corn, sugar, eggs, soy, orange and nightshades. *Serves 3-4*

1½ cups rice flakes (rolled)
3½ cups water

Place rice flakes and water in saucepan, bring to boil, then simmer till flakes are soft. Add more water if necessary. Serve with ground unhulled sesame seeds or ground almonds, a few raisins and nut milk.

Crockpot Porridge

All are free of dairy products, wheat, yeast, corn, sugar, eggs, soy, orange and nightshades. *Serves 4*

Porridge can be cooked overnight in a crockpot. Simply place grain and water in the crockpot and turn on low before retiring. In the morning the porridge will be ready.

Rice Porridge

1½ cups rice flakes
4½ cups water

Millet Porridge

2 cups rolled millet (millet flakes)
4½ cups water

Buckwheat Porridge

1 cup buckwheat
3½-4 cups water

Oat Porridge

2 cups rolled oats
4¼ cups water

Breakfast Rice Cakes

Free of dairy products, wheat, yeast, corn, sugar, soy, orange and nightshades. *Serves 2*

1 egg beaten or 2 stiffly beaten egg whites
1½ cups cooked brown rice
3 tablespoons rolled millet

Mix ingredients together. Place spoonfuls onto greased pan and flatten with back of a spoon. Cook both sides until browned and crisp. Spread with nut butter, mashed banana or a little maple syrup or honey.

Breakfast Fruit Salad

Free of wheat, corn, sugar, eggs, soy, orange and nightshades.
Can be made free of dairy products and yeast if yoghurt is omitted.

fresh fruit in season **ground nuts** **ground seeds** **goat's yoghurt or non fat yoghurt or tahini cream**	Chop fruit. Top with ground nuts and/or seeds. Serve with yoghurt or tahini cream if liked.

Sunshine Breakfast

Free of wheat, corn, sugar, eggs, orange and nightshades.
Can be made free of dairy products and yeast if yoghurt omitted.
Can be made free of soy if soy milk omitted.

Serves 1-2

1 large banana **1 thick slice pawpaw** **2-3 tablespoons fruit juice** **2 tablespoons non fat yoghurt or goat's yoghurt or pleasant tasting liquid soy milk (optional)** **1 tablespoon each of ground sesame seeds, ground pumpkin seeds and coconut**	Blend banana, pawpaw and fruit juice. Pour into a glass and top with yoghurt or soy milk if desired. Sprinkle with seeds and coconut. Serve in a parfait or champagne glass.

Pancakes and Waffles

Choose from any of the recipes in the pancakes and waffles section.
They can make satisfying breakfasts served with stewed apple, strawberry
sauce, mashed banana, tahini or nut butters.

Breakfast Sprinkle

Free of dairy products, wheat, yeast, corn, sugar, eggs, soy, orange and nightshades.

An excellent way of getting easily digested protein and natural fatty
acids is to grind up finely.

1 cup almonds **½ cup sesame seeds** **½ cup sunflower seeds** **½ cup pumpkin seeds**	Sprinkle over fruit, yoghurt or muesli.

Banana Smoothie

Free of wheat, corn, sugar, eggs and nightshades.
Can be made free of dairy and yeast if yoghurt is omitted.
Can be made free of soy if soy milk is omitted.

---

2 small bananas (e.g. lady fingers)
¼ cup orange juice
1-2 tablespoons yoghurt or pleasant tasting liquid soy milk (if using soy milk reduce orange juice)

Blend and pour into large wine glasses or a dish. Top with any or all of the following: dollop of yoghurt, passionfruit, twirl of maple syrup, coconut sprinkle.

SCHOOL LUNCHES

School lunches which are different in any way from the normal may present problems for the cook, mainly because a child may be reluctant to eat differently from other children for fear of being teased. If this is the case, homemade allergy-free breads or waffles made to look as much like sandwiches as possible may be used more successfully than something distinctly different. Below is a list of ideas which may be helpful in preparing school lunches.

Salads

Include tabouli, carrot and celery sticks, rice salad, sprouts, green salad, combined with hummus, avocado dip, pâté, nori rolls, vegetable pasties, vegetarian rolls with tomato sauce, any left over pie, pizza, loaf or rissole.

Soup

Use in winter. Pour into a vacuum flask and include bread, crackers or waffles.

Sandwiches/waffles

Make from allowable ingredients with a filling of nut butter, mashed egg, finely diced cooked chicken, avocado, tahini, hummus, curried tofu or baked beans.

Homemade muffins

Fill with a spread e.g. nut butter, berry jam, or lemon spread.

Crackers and rice cakes

Rye biscuits or rice cakes or crackers need to be filled with foods that will not cause the crackers to become soggy, e.g. nut butters.

During the summer months the lunch may include fresh fruit salad, frozen oranges or frozen fruit containers with unsweetened fruit (available from supermarkets). It is best not to send food which may become contaminated with bacteria during the warm weather, e.g. chicken, rice.

You may like to include 1 or 2 cookies, a slice of cake, fruit and nut balls or nuts and dried fruit.

PARTY FOODS

Is your child highly charged, naughty and difficult to live with after attending a party?

Parties are certainly a problem, especially for the child with allergies. Most party foods contain lots of preservatives, artificial colourings and additives as well as the major allergens — yeast, eggs, milk and wheat.

We have made a list of foods you might like to include in your child's next party, most of the major allergens and the baddies excluded.

Individual Pizzas

See recipe in Main Course section. If you wish to make individual pizzas cut out small rounds to fit into tartlet tray and fill with small amounts of pizza mix. Pizzas may be made with or without cheese.

Sesame Chicken

See recipe in Main Course section.

Sesame Fish Fingers

See recipe in Main Course section.

Stuffed Egg Boats
Free of dairy products, wheat, corn, sugar, soy, orange and nightshades.

Boil eggs until hard. Allow to cool or place in cold water for approximately 10 minutes (it is then easier to peel them). Peel eggs cutting lengthwise. Remove yolk and mash with mayonnaise and parsley or omit yolks and fill with Curried Tofu Dip. Fill cavities with mixture. Cut coloured triangular sails and mark with a number or child's name. Thread with small skewer or toothpick and insert gently into yolk mix. Serve on a bed of shredded lettuce (to resemble the sea)

Vegetarian Rolls

**Free of dairy products, wheat, corn, sugar, eggs, orange and nightshades.
Can be free of yeast if tamari is omitted.**

See recipe in Main Course Section, but cut rolls into 2-3 cm lengths.

Potato Chicken Balls

**Free of dairy products, wheat, corn, sugar, eggs and orange.
Can be made free of soy and yeast by omitting tamari.**

1½ **cups dry mashed potato** 1 **cup finely chopped raw chicken** 1½ **tablespoons finely chopped onion** 1½ **tablespoons tamari or herbal seasoning** 1½ **tablespoons finely chopped capsicum** 1½ **teaspoons chives** 1½ **teaspoons basil** **sesame seeds**	Mix together and roll in sesame seeds. Bake in a moderate oven till lightly browned. Serve in a spaghetti basket.

Spaghetti Basket

Can be made free of wheat by using corn or buckwheat spaghetti.

1 **slice seed bread** **toothpicks** **spaghetti strands (cooked)**	Toast bread. Push in toothpicks all around the edge, approximately 2 cm apart. Weave spaghetti carefully around toothpicks, turning ends inwards. Continue until reaching the tops of toothpicks. As these are very small baskets, you may need to make a few. Fill with potato straws.

Crackers with Spreads

See section on Spreads.

Festive Icecream Cake

This is an excellent substitute for the usual birthday cake. See Cakes section.

Watermelon Basket
Free of dairy products, wheat, corn, sugar, eggs, soy, orange and nightshades.

Take a whole watermelon, mark the horizontal middle line around the melon, then mark a 4-5 cm strip from the mid point of one side over to the other side. With a knife remove all of top half of melon except for this strip. Remove the rest of the flesh with a melon baller to form balls, other fruits or different melons can be added to give different colours.

Serve balls in basket.

Puffed Millet Balls
Free of dairy products, wheat, corn, sugar, eggs, soy, orange and nightshades.
Variation is yeast free.

2 cups puffed millet
¼ cup coconut
¼ cup sunflower seeds
¼ cup chopped pecans or cashews
2 tablespoons carob flour
¼ cup currants or sultanas
250 g dekama creamed coconut
1 teaspoon cinnamon
2 tablespoons honey

Combine all ingredients except honey and dekama. Melt dekama and honey over low heat, then add to dry ingredients. Roll into balls and refrigerate.

Variation:

Substitute chopped fresh dates and banana for currants.

Confectionery

See recipes in this section.

Carob/Ginger Bread Men

These can be given to take home. See Biscuits and Slices section.

Strawberries or Macadamia Nuts in Carob Cases
Free of wheat, yeast, corn, sugar, eggs, orange, nightshades and soy (unless carob block contains lecithin).

Purchase small decorative patty cases (available from some health food shops or delicatessens). Melt a block of unsweetened carob or carob buttons. Place a strawberry in the middle of each patty case and pour over melted carob.

Green Pond with Frog Jumping Out
Free of dairy products, wheat, yeast, corn, sugar, eggs, soy, orange and nightshades.

2 cups apple juice
1 tablespoon spinach juice (to colour)
1 tablespoon agar* flakes

Place juices and agar in saucepan and cook until agar has dissolved. Wet mould and quickly pour juice into mould.

    * See note on agar in glossary.

    Frog can be purchased or made from carob mould recipe — in which case you will need to purchase a frog mould.

Popcorn
Free of wheat, yeast, sugar, eggs, soy, orange and nightshades.

Melt a little ghee in a heavy saucepan. When hot add popcorn, place lid on saucepan and shake. Allow to stand over heat until all corn has popped, being careful not to burn the corn.

For a novel idea make a swagman's stick. Wrap popcorn in cellophane then in hanky and tie onto the end of a stick.

Potato Chips

See recipe in Vegetable section.

Banana with Honey and Nuts
Free of dairy products, wheat, yeast, corn, sugar, eggs, soy, orange and nightshades.

Peel banana, coat with honey and roll in chopped nuts.

Frozen Treats

Banana, Tropical Freeze and Yoghurt Pops and Frozen Carob Moulds: see Frozen Treats section.

Strawberry Sorbet

See Dessert section.

Instead of the usual bag of lollies being taken home, a small gift will avoid the sweet problem. To avoid the hassles with older children and food, perhaps a barbecue picnic may be a better arrangement than the conventional party.

BIBLIOGRAPHY

Books on allergies

Baker, Elton and Baker, Elizabeth: *The Uncook Book*. Drelwood Publications, Colorado, 1980.

Buist, Robert: *Food Chemical Sensitivity*. Harper and Row, Sydney, 1986.

Buist, Robert: *Food Intolerance — what it is and how to cope with it*. Harper and Row, Sydney, 1984.

Coca, Arthur F.: *The Pulse Test*. Arco Publishing Company, New York, 1956.

Cook, William G: *The Yeast Connection*. Professional Books, Jackson, 1983.

Mandell, Marshall and Scanlon, Lynne W.: *Dr Mandell's Five Day Allergy Relief System*. Arrow Books, Essex, 1983.

Reading, C. and Meillon, R: *Relatively Speaking*. Fontana, Sydney, 1984.

Rudolph, J. A. and Rudolph, B. M.: *Allergies — what they are and what to do about them*. Jove Publications Incorporated, New York, 1977.

Vayda, William with Smith, Jann: *Are you allergic to the 20th century?* Thomas Nelson, Melbourne, 1981.

Williams, Xandria: *Living With Allergies*. Harper and Row, Sydney, 1986.

Wunderlich, Ray C. Jnr and Kalita, D.: *Candida Albicans*. Edited by Richard A. Passwater and Earl Mindell. Keith Publishing Incorporated, Connecticut, 1984.

General books on health

Airola, Paavo: *How to get well*. Health Plus, Phoenix, 1974.

Airola, Paavo: *Rejuvenation secrets from around the world*. Health Plus, Phoenix, 1974.

Forbes, Alec: *The Bristol Diet*. Century, London, 1984.

Harrison, John: *Love Your Disease. It's Keeping You Healthy*. Angus and Robertson, Sydney, 1984.

Horne, Ross: *The New Health Revolution*. Happy Landings Pty Ltd, Avalon Beach, 1983.

Kenton, Leslie: *The Biogenic Diet*. Arrow Books, London, 1986.

Phillips, David A: *New Dimensions in Health, from soil to psyche*. Angus and Robertson, Sydney, 1983.

Pritikin, Nathan with McGrady, Patrick M. Jnr: *The Pritikin Program for Diet and Exercise*. Bantam, New York, 1980.

Wigmore, Ann: *Be your own doctor*. Avery Publishing Group, Wayne, 1982.

Wigmore, Ann: *You are your own healer*. Hippocrates Health Institute, Boston, 1979.